S. Hrg. 109–176

BACK FROM THE BATTLEFIELD, PART II: SEAMLESS TRANSITION TO CIVILIAN LIFE

HEARING

BEFORE THE

COMMITTEE ON VETERANS' AFFAIRS
UNITED STATES SENATE

ONE HUNDRED NINTH CONGRESS

FIRST SESSION

APRIL 19, 2005

Printed for the use of the Committee on Veterans' Affairs

Available via the World Wide Web: http://www.access.gpo.gov/congress/senate

U.S. GOVERNMENT PRINTING OFFICE

22–553 PDF　　　　WASHINGTON : 2005

For sale by the Superintendent of Documents, U.S. Government Printing Office
Internet: bookstore.gpo.gov　Phone: toll free (866) 512–1800; DC area (202) 512–1800
Fax: (202) 512–2250　Mail: Stop SSOP, Washington, DC 20402–0001

COMMITTEE ON VETERANS' AFFAIRS

LARRY E. CRAIG, Idaho, *Chairman*

ARLEN SPECTER, Pennsylvania
KAY BAILEY HUTCHISON, Texas
LINDSEY O. GRAHAM, South Carolina
RICHARD BURR, North Carolina
JOHN ENSIGN, Nevada
JOHN THUNE, South Dakota
JOHNNY ISAKSON, Georgia

DANIEL K. AKAKA, Hawaii, *Ranking Member*
JOHN D. ROCKEFELLER IV, West Virginia
JAMES M. JEFFORDS, (I), Vermont
PATTY MURRAY, Washington
BARACK OBAMA, Illinois
KEN SALAZAR, Colorado

LUPE WISSEL, *Majority Staff Director*
D. NOELANI KALIPI, *Minority Staff Director*

C O N T E N T S

TUESDAY, APRIL 19, 2005

SENATORS

WITNESSES

APPENDIX

BACK FROM THE BATTLEFIELD, PART II: SEAMLESS TRANSITION TO CIVILIAN LIFE

TUESDAY, APRIL 19, 2005

UNITED STATES SENATE,
COMMITTEE ON VETERANS' AFFAIRS,
Washington, DC.

The Committee met, pursuant to notice, at 10:04 a.m., in room 418, Russell Senate Office Building, Hon. Daniel K. Akaka, Ranking Member, presiding.

Present: Senators Akaka, Murray, and Salazar.

OPENING STATEMENT OF HON. DANIEL K. AKAKA, RANKING MEMBER, U.S. SENATOR FROM HAWAII

Senator AKAKA. The Committee on Veterans' Affairs will come to order.

I am very pleased to welcome all of you to this very important hearing today. Chairman Craig would be here to welcome you, however, he has an amendment on the floor this morning and will be unable to join us at this moment.

I have enjoyed working with the Chairman and know that he would be here now if he could, and we are looking forward to him joining this Committee later this morning.

I am grateful for this opportunity to talk about what the Government is doing to care for transitioning servicemembers. I echo the sentiment of George Washington from so long ago "Young people will only serve in our Armed Services if they perceive that veterans of earlier wars were appreciated by their Nation." I think these words ring especially true today. We must be doing all that we can for our soldiers, sailors, airmen and marines, as they transition from military to civilian life.

I thank all the panelists for being here today. I would like to especially welcome two of our Nation's heroes, Mr. Tristan Wyatt and 1st Lt. John Fernandez, both veterans of the current conflict in Iraq.

Mr. Wyatt grew up in New Jersey and moved to Colorado in 1998. He enlisted in the Army in October 2002, attended basic training in Fort Leonard Wood, Missouri, and became a combat engineer. After airborne school at Fort Benning, Georgia, Mr. Wyatt was assigned to the 3rd Armored Cavalry Regiment at Fort Carson, Colorado. In late February he was deployed to Iraq.

On August 25, 2003, Mr. Wyatt was wounded in action en route from Fallujah to the city of Caldiah. During the firefight, Mr. Wyatt took shrapnel and lost his right leg above his knee. He was awarded the Bronze Star and the Purple Heart on September 1st.

He arrived at Walter Reed Medical Center where he was treated until the middle of January. Mr. Wyatt was medically discharged on June 24, 2004.

First Lieutenant John Fernandez is a 2001 graduate of West Point Military Academy and was captain of the West Point lacrosse team.

During Operation Iraqi Freedom, Lt. Fernandez was a member of the Charlie Battery 313 Field Artillery based out of Fort Sill, Oklahoma. He was deployed to OIF on January 20, 2003. On April 3rd, 2003, 20 miles south of Baghdad, Lt. Fernandez was injured when a 500-pound laser-guided bomb hit in very close proximity to him. As a result of this friendly fire incident, both of his legs were amputated below the knee. Lt. Fernandez arrived at Walter Reed Army Medical Center on April 11. He was sent home from Walter Reed upon his own request on June 20, 2003. He officially left the service on August 11, 2004, 16 months after his initial injury.

Gentlemen, I look forward to hearing the testimony that you will give today. Both of you have special insight into how the Departments of Veterans Affairs, Defense and Labor systems are working. Please share your views with us so that we can better serve our newly separated servicemembers. Will both of you please move up to the desk?

I applaud the work that VA, DOD and DOL have done to ensure a seamless transition to the men and women that serve. However, the Committee needs to know if these departments are doing everything possible to guarantee that each servicemember is receiving high quality assistance. Our servicemembers, including the men and women who are coming back from Iraq and Afghanistan, should have nothing less than a seamless reintegration into society and their lives. We need to be particularly attentive to the challenges faced by the Guard and Reserves in their transition from military to civilian life.

In my own State of Hawaii more than 700 Guard and Reserve members have returned from active duty, and there are currently more than 3,200 on active duty, who will be transitioning in the future. I am very concerned that these servicemembers have the appropriate services available to them upon their return from active duty.

Again, thank you all for being here today and I look forward to your testimony.

May I call on Senator Murray for any remarks she has?

OPENING STATEMENT OF HON. PATTY MURRAY, U.S. SENATOR FROM WASHINGTON

Senator MURRAY. Thank you very much, Senator Akaka, and thank you to you and Chairman Craig for holding this hearing today, and I especially want to thank both of our witnesses for being here today.

I think how we treat our soldiers when they return home to make sure the transition back into civilian life is as seamless as possible is really critical. I think it is something we have learned from previous war experiences, certainly from Vietnam when I was younger, and as well as the first Gulf War when we discovered Gulf War syndrome, as Senator Rockefeller worked on so hard a number of years ago, that we have to listen to the soldiers who are returning and making sure that we do the best job possible.

I am hoping to have a field hearing in my home State in the future because we have thousands of Guard and Reserve returning as well.

I will submit my statement for the record, Mr. Chairman, and look forward to hearing the testimony. I have two other hearings I have to be at this morning, so I will not be able to stay a long time, but I do think this is absolutely critical. Your testimony today will help us make sure we are doing the right thing for all of the soldiers who are returning, so I really appreciate your being here today.

Thank you, Mr. Chairman.

Senator AKAKA. Thank you. Senator Murray, your statement will be included in the record.

[The prepared statement of Senator Murray follows:]

PREPARED STATEMENT OF HON. PATTY MURRAY,
U.S. SENATOR FROM WASHINGTON

I thank Chairman Craig and Senator Akaka for calling the hearing. I want to welcome the panel and thank them for their service to our country.

I have been concerned about transition issues for quite some time. They have always been a burden for the soldiers on the front lines and their families back home. I saw some of the effects of war at home when my father returned from WWII. Then, the whole country became more aware of these issues thanks to the brave men and women who came home after their experience in Vietnam. When I first joined this Committee, we were seeing the effects of a relatively short Persian Gulf War.

Now, I see the effects of this war in my visits to Walter Reed, Bethesda, my VA facilities back home, and with the families I meet all over Washington State. During my trip to Baghdad and Kuwait last month, I saw the concern in soldiers' eyes as they talked with both anticipation and trepidation about their return home. And, I hear about the concerns of returning soldiers and their families every day.

Washington State has a proud military heritage with Fort Lewis, McChord, Fairchild, and all of the Puget Sound Naval bases—each of them have sent service men and women into Iraq or Afghanistan. Fort Lewis is home to three Stryker Brigades—two have already seen action in Iraq. And, we have a large number of National Guard and Reserves who have served—or are currently in Iraq or Afghanistan. In all, over 20,000 service men and women from my home State have gone overseas in this War, and a large group has just returned. That's why I brought together the leaders of Madigan Army Hospital, our regional VA, Fort Lewis and Camp Murray last January. I wanted to know their plan to take care of the returning soldiers and their families, and to ensure they had all of the help I could provide.

Mr. Chairman, that's why this hearing is so important—we need to find out what we can do better. And we need to keep talking so more of our new veterans come forward and get the care and benefits they have earned. That's why I have asked to hold a field hearing in Washington State—because keeping the issue front and center is what my military and VA leaders have asked me to do.

Mr. Chairman, I am eager to hear from our panelists today, and review all of their testimony in the days ahead. I look forward to working with you, Senator Akaka and the rest of our colleagues on a VA benefits bill that can make our newest veterans' transitions back home as easy as possible.

I am particularly interested in the level of counseling we provide families prior to a soldier's return home. For example, do they get counseling to spot warning signs of things like PTSD? And, how can they help their loved-one adjust to life back at home, or back on the job.

I would like to hear how we maintain contact with both returning service men and women—as well as their families—during this transition period.

I am also interested in how we treat Guard and Reserve soldiers when they come back. I know there are particular challenges when many of these soldiers don't live close to military or VA facilities.

I could go on, but these are some of the issues I hope our second panel can answer for the record. Thank you Mr. Chairman, I look forward to both of our panels' instructive testimony.

Senator AKAKA. Turning now to the first panel, Mr. Wyatt, will you please give your testimony and please let the Committee know about your transition from military to civilian life.

STATEMENT OF TRISTAN WYATT,
VETERAN OF OPERATION IRAQI FREEDOM

Mr. WYATT. Good morning. I would first like to say it is an honor for me to be here today.

After wounds received in action during Operation Iraqi Freedom, I began a stint at Walter Reed Army Hospital. It lasted for 6 months of recovery and therapy.

Understanding the severity of my wounds and against my best wishes, I knew it was highly unlikely I would ever see the battlefield again. I was very disappointed, and even more, I was scared. I did not know what my next step should be or where I should go. As soon as I was coherent I found physical therapists and members of the VA began to show up at my bedside. Every day I was given information about benefits, entitlements and health care. For the most part it was overwhelming, a lot of information to take in in a short amount of time.

The thing that impressed me the most was there was always an answer to my question. I never felt blown off. They had a simple and effective way of passing the information to me in ways that I could understand and ways I could retain. This was very important.

Leaving the hospital I felt confident. I had a good understanding of what to do and where to begin once I returned home to Colorado. The process for most of my benefits and entitlements had begun at Walter Reed so when I returned it was only a matter of weeks before my benefits were in order. It was a fairly quick and effective process. The longest portion was the medical boarding. Although this was not a huge issue for me, this was a big financial and emotional setback for the soldiers who had families. It is very tough for these soldiers to wait around for months on the boarding process in order to be home with their families and begin their new lives.

On top of everything the VA has done for me and my family, they had also offered me a job recently which I accepted at the beginning of this month. It was a product of the vocational rehab process designed to give personal assistance with education, the ultimate goal is employment. This is how I was introduced to the Vet IT program at the Regional VA Office here in Washington, DC. It offers returning disabled vets the opportunity at hard-to-attain GS positions within the VA. I cannot say enough about these programs and the volunteers that run them. There were now more opportunities available to me than I could have ever imagined.

It would be great to see these programs implemented in other VA offices around the country. Many vets are not willing to move to Washington, DC because of the troubles of moving a family cross-country. This is not something that I think is wrong, but I believe we are on the verge of something very good, a great thing. I had an opportunity and was able to take advantage of it because I have no family or children to consider. I was able to move on a whim. These soldiers with families deserve the same opportunities, and more than likely they need it.

It seems to me the system is much more stressful and financially draining on the soldiers with families because of the waiting periods. From my experience and the experience of my comrades there should be more emphasis on expanding Vet IT and vocational rehab programs around the country.

My separation from the Army was made a lot smoother than expected because of people who truly care and are willing to take a chance on a busted soldier. Even though I despise the thought of leaving combat arms, my life after injury was put back on course quickly, and the result was better than I could have ever hoped for. I will forever be in debt.

It was my pleasure and my honor to fight for this great country, and I am grateful for the opportunity to work for this organization dedicated to veterans.

Thank you.

[The prepared statement of Mr. Wyatt follows:]

PREPARED STATEMENT OF TRISTAN WYATT,
VETERAN OF OPERATION IRAQI FREEDOM

I would first like to say that it is an honor to be here. My name is Tristan Wyatt. I enlisted in the Army as a combat engineer in October of 2002. After completion of basic training and airborne school I was assigned to the 3rd Armored Cavalry Regiment out of Ft. Carson, Colorado, with whom I deployed with in support of Operation Iraqi Freedom in March of 2003. During a firefight in the city of Fallujah two of my squad members and I all lost a leg on August 25th 2003. We were transported to Germany and then to Walter Reed Army hospital where I spent the better part of 6 months in recovery and therapy.

Understanding the severity of my wounds, and against my best wishes, I knew it was highly unlikely I would ever see a battlefield again. I was very disappointed and even more scared; I did not know what my next step should be. As soon as I was coherent, physical therapists begun the show up at my bedside and so did personnel from the VA. Everyday I was given information about benefits, entitlements and health care. It was often an overwhelming amount of information, but what was most impressive; there was always an answer to my question. They had a simple and effective way of passing the information to me in ways I could understand and retain. This was very important. Leaving the hospital I felt confident I had a good understanding of what to do and where to begin when I returned home to Colorado. The process for most of my benefits and entitlements had begun at Walter Reed, so when I returned home it was only a matter of weeks before my entitlements and benefits were in order. It was a fairly quick and effective process. The longest portion was the medical boarding process. Although not a huge issue for me, a single solider. This was a big financial and emotional setback for the soldiers with families. It was very tough for these guys to wait around for months on the boarding process in order to be home with their families and begin their new lives.

On top of everything that the VA has done for me and my family, they offered me a job which I accepted earlier this month. It was a product of the Vet IT program at the Regional VA office here in DC. I cannot say enough about this program and the people that run it. This program offers returning disabled Vets the opportunity at hard-to-attain GS positions within the VA IT office. Between this program and vocational rehab there were many more opportunities available to me than I could have imagined. It would be great to see this program implemented in other VA offices around the country. Many vets are not willing to come to Washington DC because of the difficulty of moving a family. This is my main concern. Not something that is wrong, but I believe we are on the verge of something great. I had an opportunity and was able to take it because I had no family or children. I was able to move on a whim. These soldiers with families deserve the same opportunities and more than likely need it. It seems to me the system is much more stressful and financially draining on the soldiers with families. From my experience and the experiences of my comrades, this should be a main focal point.

My separation from the Army was made a lot smoother than expected because of these people who truly care and are willing to take a chance on a busted soldier. My life after combat injury was put back on course quickly and the result was better than I could have ever hoped for. I will forever be in debt. It was my pleasure and honor to fight for this great country and I am grateful for the opportunity to work for this outstanding organization dedicated to veterans.

Senator AKAKA. Thank you very much.

Lieutenant Fernandez, will you please give your testimony?

STATEMENT OF 1st LT JOHN A. FERNANDEZ, (RET) VETERAN OF OPERATION IRAQI FREEDOM

Lieutenant FERNANDEZ. Good morning, ladies and gentlemen. My name is 1st Lieutenant John Fernandez, Retired. Not bad to be retired at 27. I am honored to be invited to testify about my experiences after being injured in Operation Iraqi Freedom.

I would like to first begin by thanking Chairman Craig, even though absent this morning, Ranking Member Akaka and Members of the Committee for giving me this incredible opportunity to testify.

To give you a brief background, I am from Rocky Point, New York. I am a 2001 graduate of the United States Military Academy and former captain of the Army lacrosse team. Before receiving my injuries on April 3rd, 2003, among other responsibilities I was primarily a Multiple Launch Rocket System Platoon Leader. I was married before deploying to Kuwait and will be celebrating my daughter's 1–year birthday at the end of April.

Though my military career was brief, I enjoyed every opportunity that I was given to lead my soldiers. This was especially true during my deployment to Kuwait and the ensuing invasion of Iraq. It was the culmination of years of training and hard work that gave my soldiers and I the confidence to perform like a well-oiled machine. We were thrown many obstacles, but overcame adversity in every instance.

We frequently found ourselves doing our primary job of firing rockets, but often also found ourselves doing things that we never thought that we would do as a Field Artillery Unit, such as raiding buildings, traveling across the desert providing security for downed vehicles, and pushing ourselves to points once believed out of reach. However, we never faltered and we grew as a team.

Unfortunately, after passing through the Karbala Gap and reaching about 20 miles south of Baghdad, our team took a big blow. After traveling for many hours we set up our battery and conducted security patrols, preparing to provide supporting fires for the units fighting to our north. We then prepared security shifts and started to fire rockets.

After my shift I tried to catch up on long-awaited rest. However, that was cut short when I woke up on the ground, surrounded by flames, with numbing pain in my legs. I felt for my legs, realized that they were still there. I then pulled off my sleeping bag and realized that my life had changed forever. I saw that my feet were very badly hit.

But not knowing what had occurred at the time, it was instinct to spring into action. I crawled to my HMMWV and grabbed my rifle, flak vest and Kevlar helmet. I looked for my reconnaissance sergeant in the HMMWV, but he was not there. I saw fuel spewing from the bottom of the vehicle and realized I had little time before the ammunition in the vehicle exploded. I called for my gunner, who called back to me. I crawled to his location, and after realizing the severity of his injuries, attempted to pull him away from the burning HMMWV.

That night at least five of my men were seriously injured, of which my injuries were the most severe. But more regrettably, the three men that I worked side-by-side with every day died, including the soldier that I attempted to save.

Immediately following the incident, I was medevaced to field hospitals within Iraq, then to Kuwait, and following Kuwait, to Spain. Spain was my last stop before reaching Walter Reed Army Medical Center on April 11, 2003. Throughout my journey to Walter Reed, I received good medical care, highlighted by the effort to save as much of my feet as possible. No amputations were attempted until I reached stateside. After arriving at Walter Reed I was told that I was going to receive a right below-the-knee amputation, and left symes amputation, or below-ankle amputation. The medical care that I received at Walter Reed was, in my opinion, phenomenal. The doctors cared a great deal for me, and gave my family the courtesy and respect they deserved during a time of uncertainty.

During this time my wife quit her job and left school to stand by my side. My whole family took a great amount of time off of work, and incurred the travel expenses to come visit me on various occasions. My family's lives were flipped upside down in the wake of my injuries. Luckily, there was a great amount of support, not only from my local community, but also from across America as a whole. Without the monetary help that I received from my friends and family, I would have suffered large financial losses. There was an immense amount of financial stress placed on me, and that would continue throughout my transition from military into civilian life.

Though the medical care that I received was great, there were also many difficulties that I encountered when transitioning into my new lifestyle. The Army heavily pushed for a quick discharge. However, after educating myself on the process, I knew that I could not be discharged until I reached maximum medical benefit. Facing a large pay decrease after being discharged, I had to fight to stay on active duty until I felt that I had reached "maximum medical benefit," which for me was getting as close to my prior physical condition as possible, whether that be running or whatever the case, within a reasonable amount of time. I was even told that I would receive dual compensation, or VA disability benefits and Army retirement benefits, which actually only applies to disabled retirees with 20 or more years of service.

I always conducted my own research, but my concern was how many soldiers in similar situations were enticed with incorrect information? Initially I did all of my own research. However, I have since received continued help from veteran service organizations. Without these outside veterans organizations, such as the Wounded Warrior Project, soldiers such as myself would be very lost.

And this should not be. There is an overwhelming need for precise information as injured soldiers have to negotiate through a bureaucratic process to transition into a new situation. And it is the Government's job to provide this information in an effective manner in order to facilitate the future success for injured soldiers.

I finished the medical board process 16 months after being injured, and entered military disability retirement, where I took advantage of Veterans Affairs services offered. Again, I was lucky enough to have veterans organizations help me parley the overwhelming amount of information. My wife and I are attending graduate school full time on dependent's education and vocational rehabilitation benefits respectively. I will also be using the VA grant for specially adapted housing. However, because of the financial strain of preparing myself for future employment, which is not a short process, it was necessary for me to also obtain Social Security disability benefits.

I am very grateful for all of the services that I have been provided from my Government. I never realized how great America was until I went to Iraq and saw how differently I could have been raised. I am truly proud to be an American. If I had the chance to go back in time, I would choose the same path to defend this country every single time.

This country has stood by my side and provided me with a great amount of financial help. However, I was injured in the beginning of the war, and can only hope and advocate for the same support to continue for the soldiers being injured today, because I know without the help of American society, I would have been in much more dire financial stress. However remarkable the support from society is, the question remains, should this be the job of the American people?

Again, I would like to thank you for this opportunity to testify. I would now be willing to answer questions.

[The prepared statement of Lt. Fernandez follows:]

PREPARED STATEMENT OF 1ST LIEUTENANT JOHN A. FERNANDEZ, (RET) VETERAN OF OPERATION IRAQI FREEDOM

Good morning Ladies and Gentlemen. My name is 1LT John Fernandez (RET), and I am honored to be invited to testify about my experiences after being injured during Operation Iraqi Freedom. I would like to begin by first thanking Chairman Craig, Ranking Member Akaka and Members of the Committee for giving me the incredible opportunity to testify.

To give you a brief background—again my name is 1LT John Fernandez (RET) and I am from Rocky Point, NY. I am a 2001 graduate of the United States Military Academy and former captain of the Army Lacrosse Team. Before receiving my injuries on April 3, 2003, among other responsibilities, I was primarily a Multiple Launch Rocket System Platoon Leader. I was married before deploying to Kuwait and will be celebrating my daughter's 1-year birthday at the end of April.

Though my military career was brief, I enjoyed every opportunity that I was given to lead my soldiers. This was especially true during my deployment to Kuwait, and the ensuing invasion of Iraq. It was the culmination of years of training and hard work that gave my soldiers and I the confidence to perform like a well-oiled machine. We were thrown many obstacles, but overcame adversity in every instance. We frequently found ourselves doing our primary job of firing rockets, but often, also found ourselves doing things we never thought that we would do as a Field Artillery unit such as: raiding buildings, traveling across the desert providing security for downed vehicles, and pushing ourselves to points once believed to be out of reach—however, we never faltered, and we grew as a team.

Unfortunately, after passing through the Karbala Gap, and reaching about 20 miles south of Baghdad, our team took a big blow. After traveling for many hours we set up our battery, and conducted security patrols preparing to provide supporting fire for units fighting to our north. We then prepared security shifts and started to fire rockets. After my shift, I tried to catch up on long awaited rest. However, that was cut short when I woke up on the ground, surrounded by flames, with numbing pain in my legs. I felt for my legs, realized that they were still there. I then pulled off my sleeping bag, and realized that my life had changed forever. I saw that my feet were very badly hit. But not knowing what had occurred at the time, it was instinct to spring into action. I crawled to my HUMMWV and grabbed my rifle, flak vest and Kevlar helmet. I looked for my reconnaissance sergeant in the HUMMWV, but he was not there. I saw fuel spewing from the bottom of the vehicle and realized that I had little time before the ammunition exploded. I called for my gunner, who called back to me. I crawled to his location, and after realizing the severity of his injuries, attempted to pull him away from the burning HUMMWV.

That night at least five of my men were seriously injured, of which my injuries were the most severe. But more regrettably, the three men that I worked side-by-side with everyday, died, including the soldier that I attempted to save.

Immediately following the incident I was medevaced to field hospitals within Iraq, then to Kuwait, and following Kuwait to Spain. Spain was my last stop before reaching Walter Reed Army Medical Center on April 11, 2003. Throughout my journey to Walter Reed I received good medical care, highlighted by the effort to save as much of my feet as possible. No amputations were attempted until I reached stateside. After arriving at Walter Reed, I was told that I was going to receive a right below-the-knee amputation, and left symes (or below ankle amputation). The medical care that I received at Walter Reed was, in my opinion, phenomenal. The doctors cared a great deal for me and gave my family the courtesy and respect they deserved during a time of uncertainty.

During this time my wife quit her job and left school to stand by my side. My whole family took a great amount of time off of work, and incurred the travel expenses to come visit me on various occasions. My family's lives were flipped upside down in the wake of my injuries. Luckily, there was a great amount of support from not only my local community, but also from across America as a whole. Without the monetary help that I received from friends and family I would have suffered large financial losses. There was an immense amount of financial stress placed on me, and that would continue throughout my transition from military into civilian life.

Though the medical care that I received was great, there were also many difficulties that I encountered when transitioning into my new lifestyle. The Army heavily pushed for a quick discharge. However, after educating myself on the process, I knew that I could not be discharged until I reached maximum medical benefit. Facing a large pay decrease after being discharged, I had to fight to stay on active duty until I felt that I reached "maximum medical benefit" which for me was getting as close to my prior physical condition as possible within a reasonable amount of time. I was even told that I would receive dual compensation, or VA disability benefits and Army retirement benefits. Which only applies to disabled retires with 20 or more years of service. I always conducted my own research, but my concern was "How many soldiers in similar situations were enticed with incorrect information?" Initially, I did all of my own research, however, I have since received continued help from veterans organizations. Without these outside veterans' organizations, such as the wounded warrior project, soldiers such as myself would be very lost. And this just should not be. There is an overwhelming need for precise information as injured soldiers have to negotiate though a bureaucratic process to transition into a new situation. And it is the Government's job to provide this information in an effective manner, in order to facilitate the future success for injured soldiers.

I finished the medical board process 16 months after being injured, and entered military disability retirement where I took advantage of the VA services offered. Again, I was lucky enough to have veterans organizations help me parley the overwhelming amount of information. My wife and I are attending graduate school full-time, on dependant's education and vocational rehabilitation benefits respectively. I will also be using the VA grant for specially adapted housing. However, because of the financial strain of preparing myself for future employment, which is not a short process, it was necessary for me to also obtain Social Security disability benefits.

I am very grateful for all of the services that have been provided from my government. I never realized how great America was until I went to Iraq and saw how differently I could have been raised. I am truly proud to be an American. If I had the chance to go back in time, I would choose the same path to defend this country every time. The country has stood by my side and provided me with a great amount of financial help. However, I was injured in the beginning of the war, and can only hope and advocate for the same support to continue for the soldiers being injured today. Because, I know without the help of American society, I would have been in much more dire financial distress. However remarkable the support from society is, the question remains: should this be the job of the American public?

I would like to thank you again for this opportunity to testify. I would now be willing to answer questions that anyone may have.

Senator AKAKA. Thank you both for your testimony and for being here this morning. I know you have alluded to some of the experiences you have had, but let me ask both of you, and tell you that I would like to know about each of your personal experiences in transitioning from the military to civilian life. Tell me how you found the process. Were you given appropriate and helpful information by VA and DOD? Have either of you utilized the Department of Labor's service? What did these agencies do well? What can be done better?

Lieutenant Fernandez?

Lieutenant FERNANDEZ. Sir, as I mentioned earlier, it is a lot of information to grasp as you go through the process, and a lot of times in going through that process, you get told a variety of information from just as many different people, and a lot of times that is hard to grasp, especially as you are trying to cope with a new lifestyle, the injuries that you sustained, and looking toward the future, wondering, now that my military career is over, what does the future hold for me?

So I think that it would be helpful, I guess, to facilitate the process for the flow of information. And I know that the veterans service organizations helped me do that because they were one place that I could go. They were one avenue that I could go that would give me the answers that I needed and they would send me in the right direction.

Senator AKAKA. Mr. Wyatt?

Mr. WYATT. I definitely agree with that. One of the biggest problems was just a lot of information being given at one point, and if there was a more organized manner that they could give it to you, that would definitely help the problem.

Another thing is there is a lot of waiting around going on, a lot of waiting for the med boards to happen. At that point you are still receiving Army military compensation which does not take care of a lot of the expenses, especially for soldiers with families.

A great thing that could happen is if the med board process was sped up somehow. It seems like a lot of paperwork gets lost, misplaced, and it just seems like there is a lack of organization sometimes. It really did not seem like we were prepared for the amount of wounded that were really going to come in from this war. That would definitely help the situation.

Senator AKAKA. To both of you, during the process of transitioning from active duty to the veteran status, when were you first contacted by VA? In your opinion, do you believe that it was the right time, or should it have been sooner or later?

Lieutenant FERNANDEZ. Sir, I know right away I was contacted when I was in the hospital, which was very reassuring knowing that there were people there to help me out. A lot of times initially though, a lot of that information was thrown at me, and as mentioned earlier, at certain points it became overwhelming. Over time I was able to kind of sift through the information and make sense out of it and understand where it fit into my future goals. I believe that there was a sufficient amount of help there, but the organization of that information and the way that it is presented to the soldiers when they are in the hospital might be presented a little bit easier.

Senator AKAKA. Mr. Wyatt?

Mr. WYATT. Definitely. Soon as I can remember waking up in the hospital there was someone from the VA. To say it was too early, I do not think that is accurate. I think that they should show up as much as possible. You see so many faces in the hospital, so many people are coming around feeding you information, like John said, that it is tough to even figure out who was who and who was from what organization.

What helped me the best, and a lot of my comrades over there, was to see them over and over and over again. Even if they are coming in to give you the same information, the repetition is important. You need to see that face, because there are so many people coming in to see you, whether it be doctors or press or the VA. You have to have that personal connection with them. I think that is important.

Senator AKAKA. Let me follow up before I turn to Senator Murray. Did VA contact you after their initial contact to remind you of services and programs they could provide, and when was that contact made?

Lieutenant FERNANDEZ. Yes, sir. VA did a lot of follow-up to make sure that I understood the programs that were available to me and the different opportunities that I had through the organization. I think that the repetition is important. As Tristan had mentioned, the repetition is important because you are given so much information. It was reassuring to know that the Administration was there to help out through the process.

Senator AKAKA. Mr. Wyatt?

Mr. WYATT. They contacted me as soon as I got home to Colorado from Walter Reed, and that seems to me to be where most of the wires get crossed, is when you leave the medical facility to go back home. It would be good if they had better points-of-contact from Walter Reed, so when you—I mean moving is a traumatic experience for anybody, and you are going to forget to call when you get home, so it would be good if they had plenty of points-of-contact, lots of people you can talk to when you return, but the VA did make a very good attempt at contacting me at every major transition point.

Senator AKAKA. Senator Murray.

Senator MURRAY. Thank you, Mr. Chairman.

Thank you to both of you for coming and testifying before the Committee today, and helping us understand some of what you have gone through so we can do a good job for those who are returning.

One of the concerns I have, coming from Washington State—you are from Colorado—we are a long ways away from Walter Reed. So when our soldiers return home if they have not either gone through Walter Reed and been sent out or just gone directly home, whether or not there is sufficient support services for them out there. You were at Walter Reed. You had people at your bedside every day. What have you heard from other soldiers who have just gone straight back to California or Washington or Colorado, far away from here, about their ability to get good service?

Lieutenant FERNANDEZ. Well, ma'am, as Mr. Wyatt had mentioned, the transition is a difficult one, and maintaining points-of-contact and maintaining similar information as you move, because when you move you are in most cases dealing with different representatives of the Veterans Affairs. So I know for me it was good to have a single point-of-contact through a veterans service organization that I dealt with the whole time, and they kind of helped me sift through that information, and I know that other soldiers have had problems getting the same information because in many cases they are dealing with different people. So that is an obstacle that I believe needs to be overcome.

Senator MURRAY. Mr. Wyatt?

Mr. WYATT. I definitely agree with that, as well as—I wear a prosthetic leg, and it seems to me Walter Reed is the mecca of prosthetics. They have all the new equipment. Everything is there. It gets cranked out in a timely fashion. Anytime I needed something serviced, it was immediate at Walter Reed. The biggest thing that I had to deal with was once I got to Denver they did not have all the equipment that Walter Reed did and I was not used to the process and things took a long time, and it gets frustrating.

I opted to stay at Walter Reed for 6 months because someone informed me of this. My team leader, who had arrived earlier in the same incident in Iraq, opted to go back to Colorado. I received my prosthetic leg the same time he did, and he had been in the system for a few weeks more than I had, so we were at the same progress level, but I think what stymied his process was Walter Reed and the VAs in the other States need to stay in contact with the technology and with the new products, new legs, you know, everything that goes into this prosthetic development.

Senator MURRAY. What about post traumatic stress syndrome? We are hearing a lot about soldiers who are returning, the stress situations that they are in and PTSD occurring after you have been discharged. What has been your experience with that?

Lieutenant FERNANDEZ. Ma'am, I know in my situation, from the minute I hit the hospital I adopted the attitude that I was not going to feel sorry for myself because of the soldiers that had passed away in the incident. Their families cannot say that. I think it really depends on the individual, therefore each individual needs to be assessed in a manner and they need to be reached out, and I know that was a big thing through Veterans Affairs, and they made sure that I was not undergoing any overdue emotional stress due to my injuries and situations that I might have encountered in Iraq.

So I know that that problem was handled very well from the Veterans Affairs standpoint.

Senator MURRAY. Mr. Wyatt?

Mr. WYATT. From what I have seen returning from combat, and especially if you are injured, PTSD is going to be the last thing on your mind, and to have that assessed at Walter Reed is—it is effective, but not as effective as it could be if it were assessed when you end up home with your family. PTSD is not going to be prevalent at an Army installation with a bunch of soldiers that just got back from combat. They are not going to want to go through the assessments. They are going to want to go home and see their families. They are going to want to get out of there. They are not going to want to hear it.

I think it would be much more effective to immediately assess them once they got home, before something did happen, but once they get home to their natural environment, that is when things start to teeter. I think it would be great, you know, in my instance, once I got home and I got to the Denver VA that was high on the priority list to be assessed there.

Senator MURRAY. My time is short, but I want to ask one other question. Lieutenant Fernandez, you talked about kind of pressure to be discharged. How did you experience that? Were people suggesting that you be discharged and——

Lieutenant FERNANDEZ. Well, ma'am, I think it again depends on the individual. In my case, it was not more beneficial for me to get out of the military. I was earning more of an income staying in, and as I went through the transition process I did not want to be, I guess, thrown out of the system and making less money when I had not reached what I myself determined as maximum medical benefit. For me, that was what I was running.

Senator MURRAY. Did people suggest to you that you should be discharged?

Lieutenant FERNANDEZ. I think over the past few years they have tried to speed up the process, speed up the medical board process, but again, it has to be dependent on the individual. In some cases it is not going to be beneficial for the individual soldier to be rushed out of the military, and I think it really has to be dependent on the soldiers themselves, and they need to have a say in that process.

Senator MURRAY. I appreciate both of you coming today.

Mr. Chairman, just for the record, that is one of the concerns I have. I have fought long and hard for additional funding for the VA because of the influx of the soldiers coming in and the needs that are out there.

One of the things I have heard from the other side is that these soldiers are part of the DOD system and the costs have not been put on the VA system. But I am hearing from many soldiers that they are being pushed very hard to be discharged, and as long as that pressure is there, we had better have the funding for veterans. It is one of the reasons I have fought hard for this.

I appreciate both of you being here, and I will continue to do what I can to make sure we are there for you as you return home. Thank you.

Senator AKAKA. Thank you, Senator Murray.

Senator Salazar, any comments or questions?

STATEMENT OF HON. KEN SALAZAR,
U.S. SENATOR FROM COLORADO

Senator SALAZAR. Thank you very much, Senator Akaka.

And thank you, Lt. Fernandez and Mr. Wyatt. Thank you for your service to our country. And Mr. Wyatt, since you have your roots in Colorado it is my honor to see you here and if there is ever anything that I can do for you as you move forward with the very long and productive life that you have ahead of you, I would be delighted to be at your services, as well as you, Lt. Fernandez.

Senator Akaka, I just want to thank you and Senator Craig for bringing the attention that you are bringing to this very important issue. I know that both of you have introduced an amendment to create an insurance program to help the injured servicemembers, to help their families cope with the increased burdens that they face when they face major injuries. And I am proud to work with both you and with Senator Craig on this important legislation.

We have all heard on this Committee from veterans in our States that there are a number of challenges that the VA faces in ensuring a smooth transition from active service duty to VA care. The first is simple demographics. More than 250,000 servicemembers who fought in Afghanistan and Iraq have left the military. Sometimes I think it is easy for us to forget that number, but we are talking about a quarter million lives, a quarter million members of our military services who have served there, and more than 11,000 of these troops have been injured in those operations, 11,000 people. I come from a small town that only has 840 people in the southern part of Colorado, and I can think about the sheer size of the numbers of military personnel that have been injured or wounded in both Afghanistan and Iraq. And with the kinds of injuries that these soldiers have received, it is important for us as a Nation to make sure that we are doing everything we can to provide the seamless transition between DOD and the VA.

I know that there have been problems. The VBA has had some trouble in dealing with benefits claims long before we went into war in Iraq. Though there has been some progress recently. I understand that the times for processing disability claims has gone from a high of 230 days to 160 days. When you think about having to wait in line for 160 days to have your claims processed, in my mind that is far too long. There is progress. I believe that the VBA and Veterans Administration are working on a number of different programs, but I hope that this hearing today will help us work with the VA and the VBA to make sure that we provide the best services we can to our veterans, and that we assure the seamless transition that we ought to have between DOD and the VA.

I have a more extended statement, but I will just submit that for the record, Senator Akaka.

[The prepared statement of Senator Salazar follows:]

PREPARED STATEMENT OF HON. KEN SALAZAR,
U.S. SENATOR FROM COLORADO

Thank you, Chairman Craig and Senator Akaka, for bringing needed attention to this important issue and for already taking steps to help soldiers returning home from Iraq and Afghanistan.

Senators Craig and Akaka are introducing an amendment to create an insurance program for injured servicemembers to help their families cope with the increased burdens they face. I am proud that you both worked together on this legislation and I am proud to co-sponsor it.

However, as we have all heard from veterans in our States, there are a number of challenges that the VA faces in smoothing the transition from active duty service to VA care.

The first is simple demographics. More than 250,000 servicemembers who fought in Afghanistan and Iraq have left the military. More than 11,000 troops have been injured in these operations. Many of these soldiers are returning home with missing limbs or major burns, but thousands more have wounds that are more subtle and will take years to diagnose.

The second is administrative. The VBA had trouble dealing with benefits claims long before we went to war with Iraq.

There has been some important progress recently, including reducing wait times for disability claims from a high of 230 days to 160 days. The Home Loan Guarantee Program, in particular, has seen amazing administrative successes dropping approval time from weeks to mere minutes.

However, 321,000 veterans are still waiting for disability claims decisions. Veterans have to wait an average of 8 to 10 weeks to get their GI Bill benefits. Vets who do not immediately apply to Vocational Rehabilitation are sometimes lost to the system for years.

A recent GAO report indicates that the VA has trouble anticipating its disability workload from year to year and has not fully accounted for more complicated claims stemming from war-related injuries.

The third administrative challenge deals directly with the transition from DOD to VA. VA has done a great deal to reach out to troops returning home from Iraq and Afghanistan. But there many veterans are falling through the cracks.

The VA has recognized this problem and has done its best to make it better. The VA has set up task forces and dispatched case workers to military medical treatment facilities. They have tried to reach incoming veterans earlier and better coordinate with the DOD.

These efforts have done a lot of good. As we will hear from those who have been through the system, it does work for many people. But independent analysis has consistently shown that there are still huge gaps.

The VA is having trouble getting the information they need from the DOD. The sharing of information and quality of casework management varies greatly from region to region. In some cases the DOD only gives the VA the names of new patients, with no information on severity of injury. In other cases, injured soldiers who do not apply for VA services immediately are lost to the system.

This is an administrative problem with huge implications for our fighting men and women. It is also a problem that will not be fixed with half-measures.

It is clear that the DOD needs to work more closely with the VA to share medical information. The VA also needs to redouble its efforts to fill the gaps in its outreach to make sure that seriously injured veterans are never lost to the system.

I look forward to the testimony today and to tackling this problem in a comprehensive way.

Senator AKAKA. Thank you very much, Senator Salazar.

There is currently a wealth of information available for transitioning disabled servicemembers on the Internet and through a 1–800 number. There are also the Army's Disabled Soldier Support System, the Marine For Life program, the Military One Source Program, and DOD's Military Severely Injured and Joint Support Operation Center.

Were you aware of any of these programs? And if you were aware of them, did you use them, and did you find them helpful if you did use them as a referral source or in answering those questions?

Lieutenant Fernandez.

Lieutenant FERNANDEZ. Sir, I believe the Disabled Soldiers Support System had contacted me at one time, and basically was information that I had already received. I think part of the problem lies in the fact that there are so many of these organizations, and there needs to be, I guess, a seamless amount of information, and they need to deal with the process in similar ways, because you cannot have all of these organizations operating in different directions with the same goals.

Senator AKAKA. Mr. Wyatt?

Mr. WYATT. I definitely agree. There is a lot of information coming from a lot of different sources, and they may only call one time. I got calls from a few while I was in the hospital, and it is tough to process all that information at one time and especially if they only call one time. You have no way of getting back to them. You are not quite sure even what they said sometimes. So if it could be all centralized and the information could be given in an organized manner that will cut a lot of the problems out.

Senator AKAKA. I want to thank you, Mr. Wyatt, and also to congratulate you with securing employment with VA, working on cyber security issues. I think that is wonderful when our Federal Government can hire recently separated servicemembers into the Federal workforce. Would you explain how you became aware of employment opportunities with VA?

Mr. WYATT. While I was in the hospital at Walter Reed, I was confronted with a program called Vocational Rehab. Pretty much what that does is it is really personalized testing that helps with education and employment. From there I was introduced to the Veterans IT program at the Regional VA over here. They contacted me about this program, and it helps disabled veterans acquire these hard-to-get GS position levels in the VA.

Senator AKAKA. Lieutenant Fernandez, thank you for your testimony too and your remarks, and your service to our Nation. I was very happy to see that you are utilizing the vocational rehabilitation benefits that are provided by VA too. I was additionally pleased to know that your wife is using VA benefits to get her master's degree in early childhood education. As a former teacher myself, I am very happy to see that both of you are pursuing careers in education.

What additional services do you think the Government should be providing to servicemembers and their families?

Lieutenant FERNANDEZ. Sir, I think that the education benefits and the vocational rehabilitation benefits are outstanding, and they help you through that transition period. However, as I go to full time to get my graduate degree and my wife does the same thing in the goal to transition into a new career, it becomes very difficult to obtain other employment, and there is financial stress that is incurred with that, and I think that can be addressed.

Even though there is money that is in place while you do receive educational benefits and while you do go to school, I am not sure if it is sufficient enough to be able to support a family while this is going on, especially in differing areas of the country. Costs of living differ throughout the country, and I should not be forced to live in a area where perhaps the cost of living is lower just to meet the needs of my family.

Senator AKAKA. I thank both of you for your testimony, and no question it will be helpful to us in our work in the Senate.

Senator, do you have any other questions?

Senator SALAZAR. Just one quick question, if I may, Mr. Chairman, and that is to Mr. Wyatt.

Since you went through the VA program in Colorado as I understand it, how was that experience for you, and do you have any recommendations that you might want to make to me on how we might be able to improve that system?

Mr. WYATT. The personnel and the staff you have there are a class act. I was treated like a king from the second I walked in there. You have great people. My only concern is points-of-contact. Coming from Walter Reed to Colorado there was a little bit of a discrepancy about who to contact and about what. The other thing would be the prosthetics department. They are great people down there. I think maybe with a little more funding, little bit more technology, they could really keep up with the things that Walter Reed put out. It seems like maybe a lot of the prosthetic work takes a little bit too long to get out because they do not have the proper tools to do the job.

A lot of these soldiers coming back are going to be wounded with missing extremities. There is a lot of it. I have been seeing a lot of it. A lot of my friends are missing extremities, and I think that would be a great main focus of the Denver VA. Other than that, they are doing a spectacular job.

Senator SALAZAR. We may have an opportunity if we can get moving on this new hospital out at Fitzsimmons to focus in on that particular need.

Mr. WYATT. Definitely.

Senator SALAZAR. I know you are new in the system. I guess this is a question to both Lt. Fernandez and Mr. Wyatt. One of the problems that I think we have seen in this Committee is the difficulty in the VA keeping in touch with our veterans over the long term. We recently had a GAO report that said that veterans many times do not apply for vocational aid immediately. They wait for a while to get their application, and sometimes what happens is in that gap of time the VA loses contact with its veterans. You obviously are success stories of what the Veterans Administration has done, but do you have any suggestions about how the VA can make sure it stays in contact with its veterans over the long period of time as opposed to just in the period of your injury and then the transition from DOD over to the VA system? Looking out, you are still very young men, and you obviously are going to be interfacing with the VA over a long period of time. Any suggestions on how we can assure that we keep that connectedness there?

Lieutenant FERNANDEZ. Yes, sir. I think again it is going to come down to simplifying the ways that veterans are informed about the programs that are available to them. It is a bit daunting looking at it, especially when you are coming home with these injuries and you do not know what the future holds. There is a little bit of paper pushing involved when it comes to obtaining these things, and sometimes you run into problems with when you are able to get them and there is a lack in time and you really have to stay on top of the process. That at times is a daunting task.

So if the process is simplified and information is simplified and given to the veterans to let them know exactly what they are eligible for and how they go about doing it in the most effective manner, then I think that would definitely help out the process in helping veterans get things that are going to help them in their future.

Senator SALAZAR. Mr. Wyatt?

Mr. WYATT. I definitely agree. Another thing that needs to be thought is a lot of enlisted soldiers, especially some of the ones I served with, joined the military and expected to be in there 20 years maybe as an alternative to going to college. You know, college is great. It is not for everybody. When you get discharged medically you realize that your career in the military is over, and you cannot do that. College seems a little—it seems, you know, maybe it was not what you had planned for, maybe you did not want to go right away, and they do take time to think about it. I think the VA needs just to stay in contact to make sure they are making progress, whether it be vocational rehab or a trade school or something. I think that it would be great if the VA just continually kept in contact just to make sure you are making progress, that you are not slipping through the cracks. That seems to be a big deal. People just seem to slip through and there is no contact made after a while.

Senator SALAZAR. Thank you very much.

Senator AKAKA. Thank you very much, Senator Salazar.

I want to thank our witnesses, our first panel very much for your testimony. Thank you again, because as I repeat, it will be helpful to us. Thank you.

[Applause.]

Senator AKAKA. May I at this time welcome the second panel: Admiral Daniel Cooper, who is Under Secretary for Benefits, representing the Department of Veterans Affairs; Frederico Juarbe, Jr., Assistant Secretary, Veterans Employment and Training, representing the Department of Labor and representing the Department of Defense; and John Molino, Assistant Secretary of Defense for Community and Family Policy, representing the Department of Defense.

At this time, let me call a 3–minute recess.

[Recess.]

Senator AKAKA. The hearing will be in order.

Again, I would like to welcome this panel and ask for your testimony, Admiral Daniel Cooper.

STATEMENT OF ADMIRAL DANIEL L. COOPER, UNDER SECRETARY FOR BENEFITS, DEPARTMENT OF VETERANS AFFAIRS; ACCOMPANIED BY ROBERT J. EPLEY, ASSOCIATE DEPUTY UNDER SECRETARY FOR POLICY AND PROGRAM MANAGEMENT, DEPARTMENT OF VETERANS AFFAIRS

Adm. COOPER. Senator Akaka, Senator Salazar, I am honored to be here today to discuss this very important issue of transition assistance provided to our returning servicemembers. I respectfully request that my written testimony be entered into the record.

Let me also say that I was extremely impressed as I sat here and listened to the very powerful testimony by your first panel.

Another thing I would like to do, I would like Linda Petty to stand up. Linda Petty is our representative at Walter Reed, and she is the one that has been responsible for this very good attempt at communications with all our young men and women returning. Did she stand up? I cannot see her.

Senator AKAKA. Yes, she did.

Adm. COOPER. She has done a superb job for us and she has been out there about a year now.

In the endeavor that we have here, VA works in concert with both the Department of Defense and Department of Labor. Our veterans range from returning men and women of the regular armed forces, the National Guard and the Reserve components, to those seriously disabled individuals who are case managed as they acclimate to the civilian world and the disabilities which they have received.

In response to the thousands of returning veterans from Iraq and Afghanistan, VA has taken a number of steps to ensure a smooth and seamless transition from military service to their country to the status of veterans. My opinion is that we are doing more and providing real assistance to a degree not seen before in the Department of Veterans Affairs.

In mid–2003 we recognized the need to develop case management procedures for those seriously disabled servicemembers and veterans who file a claim for disability compensation. This ensures that these individuals receive the highest level of service and all possible benefits to which they are entitled in the most expeditious and compassionate manner. For those who are not seriously injured, VBA policy does not require case management, but does require a higher-than-normal level of service, calling for direct contact and assistance in filing claims.

VBA has assigned full-time claims representatives to the Walter Reed Army Medical Center, the National Naval Medical Center in Bethesda, as well as representatives at other major military treatment facilities or MTFs across the Nation. These individuals also provide benefit counseling to seriously disabled servicemembers and their families. They serve as liaison and initiate paperwork for disability compensation claims to ensure that we have rapid processing prior to discharge and that benefits are available as soon as legally possible for those veterans.

We have OIF/OEF coordinators designated in each one of our regional offices to act as liaison with the VA medical centers, the military facilities, and other regional offices. I have tasked the regional office directors with ensuring that each one of our returning men and women are under VA control and we know where they are and what we can do for them.

Our benefits delivery at discharge, or BDD, program has continued to expand. This program facilitates the adjudication process for claims at the time of discharge. Servicemembers can file disability compensation claims prior to discharge from the military and take advantage of a significantly faster processing time once they are discharged.

VBA has significantly increased outreach efforts to all servicemembers, and particularly to those returning from active duty in the National Guard and Reserve units. VA developed and distributes pamphlets, brochures and educational videos designed for returning servicemembers, for VA employees and others involved in this important effort. These resources are utilized at various outreach events such as transition assistance briefings, benefits briefings aboard returning aircraft carriers in the last 2 years, and Guard and Reserve briefings. In fiscal year 2004, VBA conducted more than 7,200 pre-separation benefits briefings for more than 260,000 active duty attendees, and 1,400 pre- and post-separation briefings were given to 83,000 Reserve and Guard members.

Our Vocational Rehabilitation and Employment program has improved to support veterans disabled in service, to include assigning a full-time vocational rehab contractor to Walter Reed Army Medical Center. Procedures are in place at other major MTFs for counselors who can provide the service necessary to let those men and women take advantage of our Vocational Rehabilitation Programs. Vocational Rehabilitation and Employment Guidebooks were developed specifically for helping disabled servicemembers make an informed choice about the program best suited for them. And we have established important relationships with both Federal and private entities who are willing to hire injured OIF and OEF servicemembers.

The Department of Veterans Affairs has made, and continues to make, tremendous strides in service to our returning servicemembers.

I appreciate the chance to be here and I will be glad to answer any questions that you may have.

[The prepared statement of Adm. Cooper follows:]

PREPARED STATEMENT OF ADMIRAL DANIEL L. COOPER, UNDER SECRETARY FOR BENEFITS, DEPARTMENT OF VETERANS AFFAIRS

Mr. Chairman and Members of the Committee, I appreciate this opportunity to testify today on this important issue. Providing outreach to military service men and women, including Reserve and National Guard members, is a vital responsibility of the Department of Veterans Affairs (VA) and particularly the Veterans Benefits Administration (VBA). We have dramatically increased our outreach activities over the last several years to reach servicemembers, not only when they are preparing to separate or retire from the military, but also upon their induction into service and during service.

VBA is working with the Department of Defense (DOD) to ensure that all Military Entrance Process Stations (MEPS) give every inductee a copy of VA Pamphlet (21–00–1), A Summary of VA Benefits. We began providing this pamphlet to inductees in November 2004. It exposes new servicemembers to basic information about the VA benefits and services for which they will be eligible when they leave military service. We are also working with the military service departments to ensure that information packets distributed to Individual Ready Reserve and Individual Mobilization Augmentees during the demobilization process include information on VA benefits and services.

Prior to separation or retirement from the military, VBA provides much more extensive information to servicemembers on specific VA benefits and services in which they might be even more interested as they depart the military. This information is conveyed in transition briefings as part of a formal 3-day Transition Assistance Program (TAP), and during the Disabled Transition Assistance Program (DTAP), as well as during individual interviews. To further improve DTAP briefings, VBA's Vocational Rehabilitation and Employment Service developed a standardized PowerPoint presentation and a new orientation video that greatly improve the quality and consistency of our outreach briefings for servicemembers, including Guard and Reserve members.

During fiscal year 2004, VBA representatives conducted over 7,000 briefings, which were attended by over 261,000 active duty personnel and their families residing in the United States. Included were 1,400 briefings for more than 88,000 Reserve and National Guard members for whom VBA provides pre- and post-deployment briefings. In fiscal year 2005 to date, VBA has conducted just under 4000 transition briefings attended by 157,000 plus participants. Nine-hundred-seventy-four of those briefings were for over 68,000 Reserve/Guard members. Returning Reserve/Guard members can elect to attend the formal TAP Workshop as well as DTAP.

In addition to the briefings conducted in the United States, in fiscal year 2004 we conducted 625 overseas transition briefings for more than 15,180 servicemembers. Our people boarded three aircraft carriers and, during the return transit, conducted TAP briefings onboard the *USS Constellation, USS Enterprise,* and *USS George Washington* (on their return to the United States from extended deployments). To date this fiscal year, we have conducted 232 overseas transition briefings for 5,600 servicemembers, and will continue to support additional requests from the Department of the Navy for TAP briefings onboard ships.

VBA has coordinated its efforts with military officials at the major demobilization sites to ensure that VA representatives are part of the briefings provided to returning servicemembers at the time of discharge. VBA representatives work closely with personnel from VA's Vet Centers at these sites.

Soon after separation or retirement from the military, veterans, including Reserve and National Guard members called to active duty, receive a "Welcome Home Package" from VBA's Veterans Assistance at Discharge System (VADS). The package includes a letter from the Secretary, a copy of VA Pamphlet (21–00–1), A Summary of VA Benefits, and VA Form 21–0501, Veterans Benefits Timetable. A 6-month follow-up letter with similar information is also mailed to these veterans. Separate outreach mailings are sent concerning VA education and insurance benefits. In addition, the Secretary of Veterans Affairs sends a personal letter to each Operation Enduring Freedom/Operation Iraqi Freedom (OEF/OIF) veteran based on lists routinely provided by the Department of Defense. Included with that letter are VA pamphlets A Summary of VA Benefits, and A Summary of VA Benefits for National Guard and Reserve Personnel.

A VA Web page, Operation Iraqi Freedom and Operation Enduring Freedom, can be accessed from VA's home page, *www.va.gov.* Information specific to Reserve and Guard members is also included on this page as well as links to other Federal benefits in which returning servicemembers may be interested. The Web page has been accessed over 377,000 times since its activation 16 months ago.

To ensure a seamless transition for seriously injured veterans, particularly those from Iraq and Afghanistan, VBA has stationed benefits counselors to work alongside Veterans Health Administration social workers at key military installations where wounded servicemembers are frequently sent. These seamless transition counselors have been in place since 2003.

Full-time VBA representatives are assigned to work bedside with patients at both the Walter Reed Army Medical Center in Washington, DC and the Bethesda Naval Medical Center in Maryland. Part-time VBA representatives are available at five other military medical treatment facilities throughout the U.S., and VBA representatives provide service, as needed, at all other military medical treatment facilities.

As of April 5, 2005, 5,383 hospitalized returning servicemembers have been assisted through this program at the Brooke (TX), Eisenhower (GA), Madigan (WA) and Walter Reed (DC) Army Medical Centers; Bethesda Naval Hospital (MD); and the Evans (CO) and Darnell (TX) Army Community Hospitals.

In addition to our disability compensation personnel, our Vocational Rehabilitation and Employment (VR&E) Service is actively participating with other organizations to strengthen our coordination and outreach efforts to disabled veterans. The goal is to ensure a seamless transition for OIF and OEF veterans. In December 2004, VR&E conducted a briefing for 150 severely disabled servicemembers and their spouses at the Salute to America's Heroes Conference in Orlando, Florida. We are working within such service improvement workgroups as VA's Seamless Transition Coordination Office, the National Guard/VA Joint Workgroup, Army Disabled Soldier Support System (DS3) Employment Workgroup, DOD/Department of Labor (DOL) Transition Assistance Program (TAP) Steering Committee, and the Marines for Life. VBA has assigned a point-of-contact to assist the staff at the new Department of Defense Military Severely Injured Joint Operations Center in northern Virginia to assist with inquiries from servicemembers and survivors relating to VA benefits and services.

In our efforts to provide quality services to disabled veterans, VR&E has an ongoing partnership with the Department of Labor's (DOL) Veterans' Employment and Training Service (VETS). VR&E staff in 57 regional offices and more than 100 outbased VA offices work closely with DOL's Disabled Veterans Outreach Program Specialists (DVOPs) and Local Veterans Employment Representatives (LVERs) to assist job-seeking veterans. There are currently 71 DOL DVOPs and LVERs co-located in 35 VA regional offices and 26 outbased locations. Additionally, there are four VR&E personnel co-located in DOL offices in Louisville, Kentucky and St. Petersburg, Florida. DVOPs and LVERs stationed or co-located with us in VR&E field facilities have the opportunity to access the same resources available to VR&E staff. This access can help to better integrate DVOPs and LVERs into the initial vocational evaluation process with the real goal of the best delivery of employment services.

VR&E has also collaborated with DOL on training for VA case managers as well as DVOPs and LVERs. VR&E and DOL jointly produced live satellite broadcasts about the Uniformed Services Employment and Reemployment Rights Act (USERRA) and special hiring authorities for Federal employment. Originally broadcast in February 2004, the USERRA broadcast explained the law and the benefits available for veterans who desire to resume the jobs that they left when they went on active duty or in some cases, because of a disability, be reemployed with the same employer in a comparable position. This satellite broadcast has been shown over 50 times. The special hiring authorities broadcast aired in July 2004 and included information on the expedited Federal hiring process for veterans with disabilities. These broadcasts provided important information for veterans seeking employment, and copies of the broadcasts continue to be distributed to VR&E and DOL personnel across the country for use by both staff and employers. Joint efforts such as this help to ensure seamless delivery of services to veterans by both VR&E and DOL.

Additionally, VR&E and DOL have developed a draft memorandum of understanding (MOU) in which we agree to use our partnership to benefit veterans and provide quality employment services. Veterans need employment assistance as they return to civilian life and the VR&E/DOL partnership supports that need. VR&E and DOL meet regularly to discuss progress on present collaborative efforts and future possibilities.

One of our newest and most successful initiatives is our Benefits Delivery at Discharge (BDD) program. Following our outreach efforts to servicemembers still on active duty, we now have an expedited process that will enable them to file an application for service-connected compensation even before they separate from the military. The required physical examinations are conducted, service medical records are reviewed, and a rating decision is prepared prior to discharge and delivered as soon thereafter as possible. For servicemembers applying while on active duty, our goal is to adjudicate claims within 30 days from discharge. Upon receipt of the claimant's DD Form 214 (Report of Release from Active Military Service), benefits are immediately authorized and the recently separated veteran can receive his/her first disability check the month following the month of discharge or shortly thereafter. Currently, 141 military installations worldwide participate in this program. Included are two sites in Germany and three in Korea. In fiscal year 2003, we processed just under 26,000 BDD claims. In fiscal year 2004, we processed 39,000 claims. This expedited BDD process is also utilized for veterans applying for benefits within 180 days of discharge.

VA participated in a number of Family Readiness Conferences such as the Army Reserve's Annual Family Action Plan Conference. VBA, represented by the St. Louis VA Regional Office, staffed a VA benefits and services information booth along with representatives from the local Veterans Centers. It is anticipated that similar conferences will be held throughout the country. Also, local VA facilities participate in homecoming events for servicemembers returning from Afghanistan and Iraq.

Mr. Chairman, in summary, VA outreach to servicemembers and veterans is extensive and far-reaching. This completes my statement, and I will be happy to answer any questions you and other Members of the Committee might have.

Senator AKAKA. Thank you very much, Admiral Cooper.

Frederico Juarbe.

STATEMENT OF FREDERICO JUARBE, JR., ASSISTANT SECRETARY FOR VETERANS EMPLOYMENT AND TRAINING, VETERANS EMPLOYMENT AND TRAINING SERVICE, DEPARTMENT OF LABOR

Mr. JUARBE. Thank you, Mr. Chairman and Senator Salazar.

It is an honor to be here and to have been present to listen to the first panel, Mr. Chairman. It is men like Lieutenant Fernandez and Mr. Wyatt is what we are all about as America's servicemen and America's veterans, and them and their comrades in arms who stand in harm's way to defend us around the world against terrorism and to protect our freedom, so I am honored to be here.

I am pleased to update you on the efforts of this Department with respect to ensuring that our servicemembers returning home from active duty military or following activations in the National Guard or Reserve are afforded the opportunity to transition to civilian life in the most seamless fashion.

Like you, we are equally committed to providing America's veterans and transitioning servicemembers with the help they need to succeed in the 21st century workforce. We share your passion for ensuring a seamless continuum of services.

To that end we work closely with Federal, State and private sector partners in order to leverage the effectiveness of our services to both the veterans and the military community.

The Veterans Employment and Training Service is ideally structured to ensure these services are provided through its network of directors located in every State, working in close cooperation with the network of State veterans employment representatives that are provided through the Jobs for Veterans Act grants. The Transition Assistance Program is a partnership between the Departments of Labor, Defense, Homeland Security and Veterans Affairs.

Our role is to provide as many comprehensive workshops as possible, where participants learn about job searches, career decision-making, current occupational and labor market conditions, resume and cover letter preparation and interviewing techniques. Participants are also provided an evaluation of their employability relative to the job market. We offer TAP workshops throughout the United States and in Germany, the United Kingdom, Guam, Mainland Japan, Okinawa, Korea and Italy. Our goal is to provide TAP at every location requested by the armed services.

Mr. Chairman, I am sure you will agree that with regard to our recently wounded and injured servicemembers such as those on our first panel, we need to do everything we can to help them rebuild their lives.

Secretary Chao set out to do just that when she tasked my office with the creation of a program that specifically addresses the needs of our returning wounded and their families. It is called the Recovery and Employment Assistance Lifeline. The REALifeline's program is the culmination of a collaborative planning process that began in November 2003, which included the Federal Departments of Defense and Veterans Affairs, veterans service organizations, State Governments, State workforce agencies, private employers and even military service organizations like the USO. REALifelines seeks to support the economic recovery and reemployment of transitioning wounded and injured servicemembers and their families by identifying barriers to employment or reemployment, and addressing those needs as early as possible.

REALifelines has placed new specialists at Walter Reed, Bethesda, Fort Sam Houston in Texas and Fort Lewis in Washington, but its primary mission is to ensure easy access to the entire range of employment, reemployment, job training, workplace accommodation and supportive services available through the Career One-Stop Service system, and not only to the servicemember, but to the families that support them, and to spouses who have temporarily left their local jobs to be with their loved ones during recovery.

We are also a key participant in the recently established DOD Military Severely Injured Joint Support Operation Center. We have onsite at this center a full-time staff member to ensure the coordination of services provided through the public workforce system, and have just added an employer-relations liaison to coordinate direct hiring by private sector employers. Through REALifelines we have provided a practical, personal resource for servicemembers to address the biggest issue they will face outside of their recovery, their economic and career success.

The Bush Administration is deeply committed to protecting the reemployment rights of all members to the military. To this end the Department administers and enforces the Uniform Services Employment and Reemployment Rights Act, which provided reemployment rights following qualifying military service and prohibits employer discrimination against those who perform military service. Only 240,000 people and groups have been provided briefings and technical assistance on the rights and responsibilities under USERRA since September 11, 2001.

Audiences include National Guard and Reserve units, employer groups and the media. While we endeavor to brief each returning servicemember on their reemployment rights, we know that with extended mobilizations there is also a need to provide more comprehensive transition assistance. This is why we have been working with the National Guard and Reserve on providing TAP services to these returning servicemembers in many States on an informal and as-needed basis.

In summary, Mr. Chairman, the Department of Labor is working hard to improve the quality of life for veterans as well as current transitioning servicemembers and their spouses. The transition of these individuals into the civilian workforce serves to benefit the entire American labor force. Most importantly, through our efforts we express our gratitude and support for all that our military members and their families do for us.

Mr. Chairman, that concludes my statement, and I would be pleased to address any questions that you may have.

[The prepared statement of Mr. Juarbe follows:]

PREPARED STATEMENT OF FREDERICO JUARBE, JR., ASSISTANT SECRETARY FOR VETERANS EMPLOYMENT AND TRAINING, VETERANS EMPLOYMENT AND TRAINING SERVICE, DEPARTMENT OF LABOR

Chairman Craig, Ranking Member Akaka, and distinguished Members of the Committee.

It is my honor to appear before this Committee today on behalf of Secretary Elaine Chao. I would like to take this opportunity to update you on the efforts of this Department with respect to ensuring that our servicemembers returning home from active duty military, or following activations in the National Guard or Reserve, are afforded the opportunity to transition to civilian life in the most seamless fashion.

The Department of Labor is very proud of the men and women in uniform, both active and reserve, who have served in the extraordinary campaign to liberate the people of Iraq and Afghanistan and protect us as a Nation from terrorism, as well as those who have served at any other time in our Nation's history. We value their service. They were there for us when we needed them, and as Secretary Chao has said on numerous occasions, it is our turn to be there for them. We support them by providing separating servicemembers, military spouses and veterans with the help that they need to succeed in the 21st century workforce.

We are committed to connecting these men and women with employers who are very eager to tap their dedication, their talent and their skills. The Department of

Labor has many offices and programs available to help servicemembers and spouses transition more easily between job markets. Through its Employment and Training Administration (ETA), Office of Disability Employment Policy (ODEP), Veterans Employment and Training Service (VETS), or any other office within the Department, veterans, transitioning servicemembers, and their spouses remain an important focus.

VETS is ideally structured to ensure these services are provided through its network of directors located in every State, who work in close cooperation with the network of State veterans employment representatives provided through the Jobs for Veterans Act Grant.

TRANSITION ASSISTANCE PROGRAM

Since 1990, when the Department of Labor began providing TAP workshops, over one million separating and retiring military members have been given job preparation assistance. In general, servicemembers who have been on active duty for at least 180 days are eligible for TAP, and those separating due to disability are eligible regardless of the length of their active duty service.

TAP is a partnership between the Departments of Labor, Defense, Homeland Security, and Veterans Affairs. Title 10, U.S.C. Chapter 58, authorizes the Department of Labor to assist the Departments of Defense (DOD) and Veterans Affairs (VA) in providing transition assistance services to separating servicemembers and their spouses. The role of the Department of Labor is to work through VETS to conduct as many employment preparation workshops as possible, based on projections made by each of the Armed Services and the Department of Homeland Security (U.S. Coast Guard).

VETS provides comprehensive workshops where participants learn about job searches, career decisionmaking, current occupational and labor market conditions, resume and cover letter preparation and interviewing techniques. Participants are also provided an evaluation of their employability relative to the job market. Components of a TAP workshop include:
- Personal Appraisal
- Career Exploration
- Strategies for an effective job search
- Interviews
- Reviewing job offers
- Other support and assistance

Public Law 108–183 added section 4113 to Title 38, U.S.C. Chapter 41 mandating VETS to provide TAP services at military installations overseas. Before this law took effect, VETS began facilitating TAP workshops at overseas military installations where, by previous interagency agreement, the Department of Defense had provided TAP workshops since the program's inception. VETS currently offers TAP workshops at 49 sites in Germany, the United Kingdom, Guam, Mainland Japan, Okinawa, Korea, and Italy. In fiscal year 2004, 5,939 separating service personnel attended these workshops in 286 separate classes. VETS continues to expand additional overseas sites in fiscal year 2005 and beyond. Our goal is to provide TAP at every location requested by the Armed Services.

State Workforce Agency Disabled Veteran Outreach Program (DVOP) specialists and Local Veterans Employment Representatives (LVER) are the primary source for TAP workshop facilitation stateside. However, because of the distances from many of the State Employment Offices to the military installations, and to assist with the rapid growth of the program, contract facilitators and VETS Federal staff also assist with TAP.

TAP program participants receive valuable training and information that gives them an edge over other applicants for employment. TAP helps servicemembers and their spouses make the initial transition from military service to the civilian workplace with less difficulty. An independent national evaluation of the program estimated that servicemembers who had participated in TAP, on average, found their first post-military job 3 weeks sooner than those who did not participate in TAP.

Servicemembers leaving the military with a service-connected disability are offered the Disabled Transition Assistance Program (DTAP) from the VA representatives. DTAP includes about four additional hours of individual instruction beyond the normal two-and-one-half-day TAP workshop to help determine job readiness and address the special needs of veterans with disabilities.

EMPLOYMENT SERVICES AND PROGRAMS FOR VETERANS

Mr. Chairman, under the Jobs for Veterans Act (Public Law 107–288) passed in 2002, veterans receive priority in all DOL-funded employment and training programs. Separating servicemembers attending TAP may register with the workforce investment system, meaning once they are discharged and attain veteran status, they are eligible for priority in the services offered at One-Stop Career Centers nationwide.

The public workforce investment system plays an important role in meeting employers' demands for a skilled workforce. The Workforce Investment Act of 1998 (WIA) was groundbreaking legislation that sparked improvements in the delivery of employment and training services nationwide through its One-Stop delivery system. Priority of service is available to veterans in all Department of Labor funded employment and training programs, which was a significant reform under the Jobs for Veterans Act. Today, our challenge is to take those reforms a dramatic step further to promote further innovation, to strengthen the One-Stop Career Center system to better serve all workers and businesses, and to make the system even more responsive to the needs of local labor markets.

We must design a flexible workforce investment system that empowers State and local officials to create workforce solutions customized to that area's workers and employers. We must make certain that outstanding plans for innovative strategies are not thwarted by the maze of conflicting funding streams, program eligibility requirements, reporting systems and performance measures.

This approach to workforce investment is at the heart of the President's proposal for job training reform. The centerpiece of the President's proposal is the consolidation of the WIA Adult, WIA Dislocated Worker, WIA Youth, and the Employment Service funding streams into a single grant to States. Governors would have the option of including an additional five programs, including Veterans Employment programs, into that single grant. Together, these programs represent over $7.5 billion in Federal resources. The consolidated grant would have a single State Integration Plan and a single performance and reporting system, thereby simplifying planning and reporting requirements. While program-specific requirements will be minimized, drops in participant levels for targeted populations, such as veterans, will not be allowed. In addition, the veterans' priority of service provision that applies to all DOL-funded programs will continue to apply, consistent with the Jobs for Veterans Act.

RECOVERY AND EMPLOYMENT ASSISTANCE LIFELINES (REALIFELINES)

Mr. Chairman, I am sure you will agree that everyone who visits wounded soldiers—whether at Walter Reed, at Bethesda, or other military hospitals around the country and around the world—comes away with an overwhelming sense of pride, humility, and gratitude for the courage that these young men and women display as they confront the reality of their injuries. In these hospitals, many efforts are underway to do everything possible to help these wounded warriors recover from their injuries. And the Department of Labor recognizes that we too need to do everything we can to help them rebuild their lives.

Secretary Chao set out to do just that when she launched a new program last October at Walter Reed Army Medical Center. It is called the Recovery and Employment Assistance Lifelines or "REALifelines" Program.

The REALifelines program is the culmination of a collaborative planning process that began in November 2003 and has included participation from the Federal Departments of Defense and Veterans' Affairs, State governments, State workforce agencies, veteran service organizations, private employers and even military service organizations like the USO. This program was built from the ground-up by service providers, by disabled veterans and even veterans of the Gulf War and Operation Iraqi Freedom. The purpose of REALifelines is to provide wounded and injured servicemembers and their families with personal assistance to ensure a successful transition to civilian life and to prepare them for rewarding careers. In addition to assisting wounded and injured servicemembers, REALifelines makes job training and employment services available to spouses in families that have suffered an active duty casualty, as well as to family members who have temporarily left their jobs to be with their loved ones during recovery.

REALifelines representatives are currently stationed at Walter Reed Army Medical Center and Bethesda National Naval Medical Center, and new specialists have begun work with the 654th Medical Holding Company at Fort Lewis, Washington, and Fort Sam Houston in San Antonio, Texas. REALifelines representatives are State workforce system employees with experience in career coaching, case management, job searches, transition assistance, reemployment rights and crisis intervention. And because they are an integral part of the State workforce system in which that base or holding company is located, they have full knowledge of, and access to, One-Stop Career Center Services, and become powerful advocates for priority of service. We are in the process of placing these employment representatives at additional military medical centers and medical holding companies.

The Department of Labor is also a key participant in the recently established DOD Military Severely Injured Joint Support Operations Center. We have onsite, a full-time REALifelines staff member to ensure the coordination of the full array of employment and training services provided through the public workforce system, and have just added an employer-relations liaison to coordinate direct hiring by private sector employers. As you know, the Joint Center is also partnered with the Transportation Security Administration to ensure that those severely injured traverse our Nation's airports in a safe, respectful and non-invasive manner.

The most important aspect of this program is person-to-person assistance. In an age where web and online utilities and technologies are gaining dominance over human interaction, it is our belief that there is still no substitute for direct person-to-person relationships—face-to-face as much as possible—when assisting people and families struggling with the challenges of wounds, injuries, crisis and post-traumatic reintegration. Therefore, the first task of REALifelines representatives is to establish for the servicemembers and their family a personal contact in their hometown community with whom they can begin to plan for their recovery and reemployment even before they are discharged from the military service. The REALifelines program looks first to the resources at hand, builds efficiency within those systems, and then works actively to fill gaps where they exist.

The greatest challenge we face is that of information collection and sharing. At present, we are tracking servicemembers through their voluntary enrollment in State employment systems and through follow-up calls made by the Job Accommodation Network, which has been operating a demonstration program to facilitate referral, outcome measures and problem resolution.

Our goal in partnership with DOD and Veterans' Affairs is to establish a joint database and shared processes for tracking and reporting outcomes. For this reason, we have placed staff at the Joint Operations Center and circulated recommendations for joint data elements both for servicemember employment profiles, and for job information from hiring employers. Labor participants are working daily with employment focused working groups from the Joint Operations Center and the Army's Council of Colonels, which provides policy and leadership for the Disabled Soldier Support System. Our goal is to be able to share this valuable data at the Federal level.

REALifelines is about closing the gaps between Federal, State, local and private systems. It is about creating greater efficiency, being proactive, and assuring responsiveness to the needs of our returning wounded and injured servicemembers and their families. Our early successes are proving the value of this program. We are reducing the number of servicemembers returning home without jobs and we are reducing the number of servicemembers losing their jobs upon return. We have provided a practical, personal resource for servicemembers to address the biggest issue they will face outside of their recovery—their economic and career success.

New initiatives are being developed in partnership with DOD and the VA, such as mentorship and Federal internship opportunities. The Department of Labor intends to be a model in Federal hiring, and in the provision of mentorship opportunities for servicemembers during their recovery. We believe that opportunity is a very powerful and effective tool for recovery and reintegration.

NATIONAL GUARD AND RESERVE

Mr. Chairman, the world has changed dramatically since the attacks of September 2001 and the commencement of the Global War on Terrorism. Our worldwide military commitments have necessitated a mobilization of National Guard and Reserve members that is unprecedented in modern times.

The use of the National Guard and Reserves has increased dramatically in recent years, with more called to active duty than at any other time since the Korean War. Over 485,000 men and women of the National Guard and Reserve components have been called to active duty since September 2001. Over 310,000 of these "citizen-soldiers" have returned and been demobilized or separated from the military. The Bush Administration is deeply committed to protecting the reemployment rights of the Guardsmen and Reservists who so bravely serve America in Iraq, Afghanistan and around the world. To this end, the Department administers and enforces the Uniformed Services Employment and Reemployment Rights Act (USERRA), which provides reemployment rights following qualifying military service and prohibits employer discrimination against those who perform military service. The Department of Justice and the Office of the Special Counsel also provide USERRA enforcement services.

Our servicemembers deserve the peace of mind that comes with knowing that upon their return from military service, they will be entitled to prompt reemployment in the position that they would have held had they been continuously employed by the civilian employer during their period of service, or in some cases to a comparable position, including all attendant benefits. Our strong commitment to supporting our citizen-soldiers is underscored by the development, for the first time, of comprehensive regulations on USERRA. These regulations will provide an authoritative interpretation of the law and procedures for enforcement and will serve to improve USERRA compliance. The proposed regulations were published for comment in the *Federal Register* on Monday, September 20, 2004, and it is anticipated that final regulations will be published this year.

Since the attacks of September 11, 2001, the Department of Labor's Veterans' Employment and Training Service (VETS) staff has conducted briefings and provided technical assistance to over 240,000 people and groups on their rights and responsibilities under USERRA. Audiences include National Guard and Reserve units, employer groups, and the media. While we endeavor to brief each returning servicemember on their reemployment rights, we know that, with extended mobilizations, there is also a need to provide more comprehensive transition assistance.

As a result, we have been working with the National Guard and Reserve on providing TAP services to these returning servicemembers in many States on an informal and as-needed basis. However, recently we launched three formal Reserve Component TAP demonstration programs in Oregon, Michigan and Minnesota, where there was a compelling need for these workshops. The idea behind the Reserve Component TAP demonstrations is to work with returning units and provide a flexible format that allows for a tailored transition assistance package that meets local demands. The approach in each location is unique. Once we evaluate the success of these programs and review any feedback from participants, we will work with the National Guard Bureau and Office of the Chief of Army Reserve to create flexible models that can be adapted to fit any situation.

EMPLOYER OUTREACH AND THE PRESIDENT'S NATIONAL HIRE VETERANS COMMITTEE

The Jobs for Veterans Act established the President's National Hire Veterans Committee, which was announced by Secretary Chao in February, 2004. There are 21 members who are reaching out to employers to make veterans more visible in our 21st century workforce.

This Committee is responsible for raising awareness among employers on the advantages of hiring veterans and transitioning military members. Last year, the Committee launched a national campaign designed to drive employers to One-Stop Career Centers and to reinforce the outreach efforts of our LVERs and DVOPs. The Committee has also reached out to Governors, and to date, 30 gubernatorial proclamations have been announced declaring HireVetsFirst months in their respective States. We expect all States will announce these proclamations by the end of fiscal year 2005. The Committee has also forged significant strategic partnerships with major American businesses and corporations.

The message of this campaign is simple; it is good business to hire a veteran, and it's a message the President's National Hire Veterans Committee is carrying all across America to employers and veterans.

PARTNERSHIP WITH DOD

On July 11, 2003, the Secretary of Labor and the Secretary of Defense signed a Memorandum of Understanding (MOU), which directs the Departments to study and undertake activities of mutual interest that may expand recruitment, job search services, training, placement, licensing and certification, and other services for military personnel, veterans, and their families. Under the MOU, work has focused in three key areas—recruitment, retention, and reentry. VETS, along with other key agencies in the Department of Labor, has fully participated in this collaboration, which has resulted in a wide array of new and/or enhanced strategies for serving these audiences.

An area of particular focus in which VETS played a key role is enhancing the connection of transitioning military personnel to One-Stop Career Centers through the TAP program. For example, one of the products has been a supplement to the TAP manual providing detailed information about One-Stop Career Center services and how to access them.

In addition, the Departments are working on a compilation of successful partnering strategies now employed by TAP staff and One-Stop Career Centers in the field. This guide to best practices will soon be distributed to TAP offices and the workforce investment system nationwide.

The goal of these efforts is to educate program staff about the benefits and commitments involved in local partnerships and encourage them to leverage their resources. Direct business connections to TAP workshops are constrained by the mandated curriculum and limited time of the TAP workshops. However, promoting ties between the TAP offices and One-Stop Career Centers generally will help separating service personnel connect with businesses.

The impact of these changes to the existing TAP program and workshops as well as the education and encouragement of local partnerships between TAP and the workforce investment system will ensure that transitioning military personnel are aware of and utilize all of the resources available to them as they search for employment and training opportunities.

NATIONAL EMERGENCY GRANTS FOR MILITARY SPOUSES

The Department of Labor has also established a policy that States may apply for National Emergency Grant funds to enable the spouses of returning Guard or Reserve members, widows of military personnel who lost their lives on active duty, and certain other military spouses, to be provided employment and retraining assistance.

SUMMARY

In summary Mr. Chairman, the Department of Labor is working hard to improve the quality of life for former, current, and transitioning servicemembers and their spouses. The transition of these individuals into the civilian workforce serves to benefit the entire American labor force. Most importantly, through our efforts, we express our gratitude and support for all that our military members and their families do for us.

Senator AKAKA. Thank you. Thank you very much.

Mr. John Molino.

STATEMENT OF JOHN MOLINO, DEPUTY UNDER SECRETARY OF DEFENSE FOR MILITARY COMMUNITY AND FAMILY POLICY, DEPARTMENT OF DEFENSE

Mr. MOLINO. Mr. Chairman, Senator Akaka, Members of the Committee, thank you for the opportunity to discuss the Defense Department's commitment to and effort on behalf of our severely injured servicemembers and their families. Thank you too for presenting the forum that allows, on behalf of the Department and everyone serving in the global war on terror, to thank our Nation's citizens for their strong, consistent and sincere support of the men and women who risk so much to protect freedom.

Each military service has an active program appropriate to the number of severely injured within that service. The Military Severely Injured Joint Support Operations Center was established to make a long-term commitment and to fill the gaps and seams that may exist in individual service programs. It reaches beyond the Department of Defense to other Government agencies, the nonprofit world and corporate America.

In addition to helping solve immediate problems, the Center will identify challenges that require systemic, policy or legislative solutions for this and future conflicts. We have adopted a case management approach that we call "care management." Highly qualified individuals, nurses or licensed social workers, answer the toll-free phones when they ring. In addition, we are using information provided by the Army to reach out to those who may have already passed through the system to ensure that their needs are being met.

For many, we are about easing the rehabilitation and return to active service. For those whose service in uniform was truncated by the injuries they sustained, we want their transition to civilian life to be as free of complications as possible. If the bureaucracy must be fought, we will fight it. If corporate America must be reminded of its obligation to help find these talented citizens a new career, we will remind its leaders. Often the spouse must become the primary wage earner. We will help in that regard as well.

Additionally, we will help those communities across America that are prepared to embrace one of these returning heroes to guarantee that he or she will never spend a holiday alone, will never want for meaningful employment, will never be left to wonder if America has forgotten.

The Center is a living entity that will be in existence for as long as it takes. Its structure may change. Its roles may be modified to ensure it remains relevant, but our commitment to the severely injured and their families is solid and long term.

Service in uniform is a noble undertaking. All who serve have volunteered. Each is deserving of our respect and admiration. All must be able to serve with the knowledge that the Congress, the Department of Defense and the Nation will neither forget nor abandon them should they suffer a traumatic injury in the service of freedom and the Nation that best represents freedom in the world.

I welcome the opportunity to respond to your questions.

[The prepared statement of Mr. Molino follows:]

PREPARED STATEMENT OF JOHN MOLINO, DEPUTY UNDER SECRETARY OF DEFENSE FOR MILITARY COMMUNITY AND FAMILY POLICY, DEPARTMENT OF DEFENSE

Mr. Chairman and Members of this distinguished Committee, thank you for the opportunity to be here today. It is my privilege to discuss the transition assistance provided to separating members of the armed forces, particularly those who have sustained severe or debilitating injuries in the line of duty.

Congress deserves sincere thanks for its continued support of our efforts to ease the transition from military to civilian life for all our separating men and women in uniform. Your interest and assistance on this matter, both individually and as an institution, are very much appreciated.

SEVERELY INJURED

I will focus this testimony on the actions taken to assist our severely injured as they reintegrate into their hometowns across America. These troops and family members who sacrificed so much deserve nothing but our best effort to assist them on their return to civilian life. Each of the Services has initiated an effort to ensure that our seriously wounded servicemembers are not forgotten—medically, administratively, or in any other way. To facilitate a coordinated response, the Department has established the Military Severely Injured Joint Support Operations Center. We are collaborating, not only with the military Services, but also with other departments of the Federal Government, nonprofit organizations, and corporate America, to assist these deserving men and women and their families.

A number of our severely injured servicemembers will be able to return to duty, thanks to their dedication and commitment, and the phenomenal quality of military medicine. Some, however, will transition from the military and return to their hometowns or become new members of another civilian community. These are capable, competent, goal-oriented men and women—the best of our Nation. They represent all the components bravely serving our Nation—the active ranks, the National Guard and the Reserve. We will ensure that during their rehabilitation we provide a "case management" approach to advocate for the servicemember and his or her family. From the Joint Support Operations Center here in Arlington, Virginia, near the seat of Government, to their communities across America, we will be with them. This will continue through their transition to the Department of Veterans Affairs, and the many other agencies and organizations providing support to them. Our goal is to provide long-term support to ensure that no injured servicemember is allowed to "fall through the cracks."

I have mentioned that the Joint Support Operations Center is a collaborative effort, both inside and outside the government. I recognize and appreciate the interest and expressed desire of the Congress to help ensure the success of this effort. As we identify the need for statutory changes, we will be certain to make you aware and seek your assistance.

The Center continues to provide a central point-of-contact for information and support through a toll-free hotline, available 24 hours a day, 365 days a year. Families are a primary focus. Since the Center's grand opening eleven weeks ago, our staff of care managers has fielded in excess of 1000 calls from injured personnel, their families or caretakers, and has placed in excess of 1000 calls in outreach efforts to find those same families who may have gone unnoticed or may require assistance. The contact numbers are growing. Callers reach the center with questions and concerns on topics that include immediate financial assistance, family support, lost promotion paperwork, employment after discharge, and healthcare. VA benefits and services remain the areas of greatest concern. Each new question or difficulty our staff is asked to address helps us to improve the service and may provide an opportunity for systemic improvements.

We remain committed to helping wounded servicemembers reintegrate into their hometowns. Moving forward, the center will seek to provide avenues to improve assistance with job placement and assistance, non-medical counseling, and financial support. We are also eager to do more for the spouses of injured personnel—who often become the primary breadwinners, or face career difficulties as they cope with the difficulties of the reintegration process.

Of course, only a coordinated, multi-agency effort will ensure that those severely injured servicemembers and their families who return to civilian life, receive the level of care and access to resources that they deserve. Through the Joint Support Operations Center and other programs and initiatives, the Department of Defense has partnered with the Department of Veterans Affairs, the Department of Labor, the Department of Homeland Security, corporate America, and various levels of government to help ensure the myriad needs of our severely injured are met. Particularly successful has been the Center's relationship with the VA in addressing and resolving specific VA benefits and health entitlement issues and concerns. We communicate through a hot-line for emergency VA issues requiring immediate VA attention, and using special e-mail address to communicate non-emergency issues. In these instances, the VA has committed to a 24-hour turnaround. The Center has been able to facilitate the rapid resolution of many issues. The Department of Labor is assisting us in obtaining civil service and private sector jobs through its One-Stop Career Centers around the country and we are working closely with the Recovery and Employment Assistance Lifelines (REALifelines), which was announced by Secretary Elaine L. Chao on October 4, 2004. Similarly, to ensure facilitated and dignified security screenings of our severely injured as they travel through our Nation's airports, the Transportation Security Administration has stationed watch standers at the Center to do just this. When the Center receives word that a severely injured servicemember will be flying domestically, the TSA team will contact all airports on the itinerary to alert the appropriate offices at these locations. Not only have TSA folks around the country prepared for the expedited screening of these travelers, they have treated them like the heroes they truly are.

The DOD State Liaison office is also actively engaging with State and local legislatures to rally communities and help guide their efforts in support of not only the severely injured, but all in-state military members and their families, to include the National Guard and Reserve. The office will be participating in the National Governors Association conference later this month and will be discussing many of these issues.

SERVICE SUPPORT FOR THE SEVERELY INJURED

The center, of course, would be nothing without the individual service and community efforts it coordinates. The centralized call center is designed to augment service programs, ensuring that, true to tradition and established practice, the Army, Navy, Air Force and Marine Corps are able to take care of their own.

MARINE FOR LIFE

The Marine Corps, building on the organizational network and strengths of the previously established Marine for Life Program, has implemented an Injured Support Program to assist severely injured Marines after they are discharged. The goal is to impress on them that the Marine Corps will always be there for them and to help them bridge the often difficult and lengthy gap between military care and the care provided by the Department of Veterans Affairs. The key is to ensure continuity of support through their transition. Features of the program include advocacy within the Marine Corps and Navy for the severely injured and their families and assistance in getting over the hurdles of any external agencies with whom they interact. Other extremely important features are pre- and post-service separation case management, assistance in working with physical evaluation boards, and an interactive website for disability/benefit information. To improve Department of Veterans Affairs handling of Marine cases there is a Marine liaison officer embedded within the VA headquarters. The program began operations in early January.

ARMY DS3

On April 30, 2004, the Army established the Disabled Soldier Support System (DS3) initiative to provide its severely disabled Soldiers and their families with a system of advocacy and follow-up with personal support to assist them as they confront the stress of their wounds and to think through the difficult decisions of continuing to pursue a military career or transitioning to the civilian community. Working closely with the Joint Support Operations Center, DS3 incorporates and integrates several existing programs to provide holistic support services for severely injured Soldiers and their families throughout their phased progression from initial casualty notification to their return home and departure from the Service. The system facilitates communication and coordination between severely injured soldiers and their families and the pertinent local and national agencies and organizations, such as the Department of Veterans Affairs and the many commendable veterans service organizations. In addition, DS3 utilizes a system to track and monitor severely disabled soldiers for a period of up to 5 years beyond their medical retirement in order to provide appropriate assistance through an array of existing service providers.

AIR FORCE PALACE HART

If an Air Force servicemember is wounded in action, the Air Force is committed to do whatever it takes to help them recover. Their Palace HART (Helping Airmen Recover Together) program follows Air Force wounded in action until they return to active duty, or are medically retired. It then provides follow up assistance for 5–7 years post injury. The Air Force works to retain injured servicemembers on active duty if at all possible; however, if unable to return an Airman to active duty, work to get them civilian employment within the Air Force. The Air Force also ensures counseling is provided on all of the benefits to which an individual servicemember may be entitled within the Department of Defense, Department of Veterans Affairs, and Department of Labor.

NAVY SUPPORT FOR THE SEVERELY INJURED

The Navy has a coordinated and tailored response for its men and women returning from Iraq, Afghanistan and other areas of conflict with severe debilitating injuries. These servicemembers, and their families are faced with very difficult long-term challenges, and the Navy team provides a strong, coordinated and unified approach to assist them and their families to recover and reintegrate.

NATIONAL SUPPORT

The response from corporate America to our severely wounded veterans has been extremely positive. Many companies including those in the Fortune 500 have opened their arms to welcome the severely wounded into their companies through direct employment opportunities or internships for gaining invaluable experience and training. Corporations can post jobs on *Military.com* for the severely injured or their spouses (*Military.com/support*). We are also developing an Adopt a Service Member program to enable communities, corporations, businesses, and even private citizens to sponsor severely injured servicemembers and their families to help them with their respective needs.

Academia has been similarly supportive of our efforts. The Department has been approached by colleges and universities interested in honoring personnel wounded in Iraq and Afghanistan. Some, like Ferris State University, are lowering their tuition charges for the severely wounded. Others, like Central Texas College (CTC), are developing special scholarships for the brave men and women who have been wounded. CTC has established twenty full scholarships, the CTC Iraqi Freedom Scholarship, for wounded personnel or for the spouses and dependents of those wounded or killed in action. Other institutions are stepping forward to help as well.

We are establishing a web presence that will encourage and allow institutions from across the country to be placed on a list of schools that want to help in this regard. That site will be linked to website hosted by the Voluntary Education program, the Transition Assistance Program, and other agencies.

TRANSITION ASSISTANCE FOR ALL THOSE LEAVING THE MILITARY

As you know, the Department and Military Services provide outstanding transition assistance to both Active and Reserve Component servicemembers. Upon demobilization, Guard and Reserve members, like their counterparts in the Active Component, receive the mandatory pre-separation counseling. The pre-separation briefing explains the transition benefits and services that they are entitled to receive as a result of their service. Topics covered include employment, relocation, education and training, health and life insurance, finances, and disabled veterans benefits.

With the support of our partners from the Departments of Labor and Veterans Affairs, we provide each Reserve Component servicemember a Uniformed Services Employment and Re-employment Rights Act briefing as well as a VA benefits briefing. These are in addition to the mandated pre-separation counseling briefing.

In conclusion, on behalf of our servicemembers and their families, thank you to the Committee for your support during these demanding times and thank you for the opportunity to thank the Nation for the support of its citizens for the noble service of America's sons and daughters.

Senator AKAKA. Thank you very much. This is the second hearing that this Committee has had on the issue of seamless transition. We heard at the first hearing and again this morning that information needs to be provided in a more organized manner, particularly for soldiers recovering from injuries. What kind of coordination and processes can your agencies utilize to address this concern?

I want to ask Admiral Cooper: Several newspaper accounts have chronicled the plight of returning servicemembers who had to overcome obstacles to undertake their studies including the lack of timeliness in getting funds from VA to the veteran; in articles, Jack McCoy, Director of the VA Education Service said that an influx of veterans going to school with the VA's help, too few claims processors and a computer glitch are among the reasons for the backlog. The fiscal year 2006 budget includes a decrease of 14 education claims processes.

My question to you is how has this impacted the current situation?

Adm. COOPER. I would say that we are overcoming the problems identified by Mr. McCoy. We have assigned a few more people to help in processing education claims. We are, however, pretty much inundated by claims coming in, rightfully so. Education claims are up about 10 percent each of the last 3 years and part of the reason for that is the things that Congress has done to enhance the Montgomery GI Bill, making the education program more desirable to returning veterans.

So we have had a larger influx. We have increased the number of people and we are watching the workload very carefully. I would say to you that, in fact, even today although we are not to our targeted goal, we are about 10 days to 2 weeks better in the processing of the education claims than we were 3 years ago. So whereas we have made progress over the years, we are not yet where we want to be. There are a few glitches now and then, and we resolve them as soon as we find out about them.

Senator AKAKA. Secretary Molino, DOD recently established the Military Severely Injured Joint Support Operations Center. The Army has its Disabled Service Members Support System, the Marines have the Marine for Life Program, the Air Force has its Helping Airmen Recover Together program, and the Navy is working on its Injured Marine and Sailors Initiative. What is being done to ensure that these programs are coordinated with each other and with the VA?

Mr. MOLINO. Senator, the establishment of the Joint Support Operations Center is in part to address the need to ensure that there is collaboration, that there is coordination. The services are each stressing different features of their individual assistance programs. They do some parts better than others. The Joint Support Operations Center enables us to share best practices, enables the services to adopt those best practices of perhaps another program that they may not have thought of. It also allows us to identify opportunities where it is best to centralize and it is best for the Joint Support Operations Center to be the primary provider of a degree of support.

As I said in my oral statement, we realized that there were gaps and there were seams between the services that should be provided, the needs of the servicemembers and the ability of our programs to provide those services. So the Center is either an umbrella or a safety net depending on how you prefer to look at it, to ensure that we fill those gaps and seams. It extends as well to the other governmental agencies, the VA and Department of Labor are noteworthy here, but we have also coordinated with Transportation Security Administration and other agencies to ensure that there is collaboration and there are ways to help.

Seamless transition between DOD and VA has been a problem and a daunting issue for many, many years, as you know from your long service in the Senate, sir. We are working as diligently now as we have ever worked. Certainly the need is more apparent now than perhaps it ever was. I know that the Department of Defense is committed, and I am fully confident, based on Admiral Cooper's comments and our experience working with the VA, that we are committed to working out whatever seams remain, working through the administrative hassles. If there are any statutory hassles, we will work through those as well with your collaboration and cooperation to do the best we can for our deserving heroes.

Senator AKAKA. And the process, is DOD establishing a DOD-wide standard for these programs?

Mr. MOLINO. We have not done that, Senator, and I think that may materialize at the end of the Joint Support Operations Center. We are trying to present the center as something that enables the service programs to succeed. The feedback we have received from many of the injured veterans, and frankly, the testimony this morning will be very helpful because it presents a different perspective that I had not heard.

We have heard from injured Marines, for instance, that they want to be helped by Marines. They want to know that the Marine Corps was with them from beginning to end. The Joint Support Operations Center is intended to allow the Marine program to succeed. If we need to fill in something that they perhaps do not have the resources, the funding or the equipment to do, we are happy to do that. But when that Marine goes home and he looks back on his service and he or she is trying to influence a young high school graduate about whether or not he or she should serve, we want them to be able to say, "The Marines were with me from beginning to end."

So while it may seem redundant to have individual service programs, we do think it is important. We will stay in the background. The name of the center is particularly awkward, I will have to admit, but it is almost by design that way. It does not reduce itself to a fancy acronym. If a Marine wants to know who helped him, it is Marine for Life. If an Army soldier wants to know who helped him, it is DS3. I am fine with that. We will stay in the background. We just want to make sure that none of the service programs ever fail.

And, Senator, if I could indulge you just one more brief period of time, I failed in my oral statement to mention the toll-free number, and since I know that this is being recorded and there is a likelihood that it will be broadcast, I would like to say that the toll free number for the Joint Support Operations Center is 1–888–774–1361, and for anyone who hears this, who knows of an injured servicemember or a family member who is worried about that servicemember, we can be the start point. We will be the warm referral either to the VA, to Labor or to the services to make sure that happens.

Senator Murray mentioned post traumatic stress disorder. We are beginning to see, we think, some of that come forward. And as you know, post traumatic stress disorder sometimes waits a decade before it manifests itself. If a family member sees any signs of PTSD, a phone call to the center will begin that support to help a veteran who may be suffering from PTSD.

Senator AKAKA. Thank you. With this wide array of programs that we are talking about, what are they doing to educate separating disabled servicemembers of where they should turn? Strangely it seems that there is competition among the services rather than coordination and synchronization. You mentioned redundancy too. What is being done to prevent this?

Mr. MOLINO. There is always some healthy competition, Senator, and where it is healthy I won't interfere. But what we have seen in this instance is an enormously high degree of collaboration. We have seen the services step forward. If a Marine goes home to an area where there is no real Marine presence, but there is an Army presence, the Army program with a regional coordinator has stepped forward to be of assistance.

We are trying to, as I said, be the collaborative point so that the support can be rendered in that fashion. But I have seen more collaboration than competition. One thing that both John and Tristan mentioned at the first panel is the flow of information that happens even while they are still patients. The truth of the matter, Senator, is they are drinking from a fire hose. There is no way we can expect them to absorb all that information immediately.

I have had the privilege of meeting with injured servicemembers while they are in the hospital. Their heads are still very foggy. Very often they are still on pretty serious medication. They cannot be expected to comprehend all of this the willingness of the Departments of Labor, Veterans Affairs and Defense, the presence of the Center. When they get home or when their heads clear, any hour of the day or night—this is a 24/7 operation—they can make a phone call and say, "I didn't quite understand what I heard," or "This is what I think I heard. Is that true?" The Center can be that first step to clearing away the fog that is understandable when they first got a piece of information, and help them to get the help or the assistance they need.

These are great Americans who are going to live great and productive lives, and it is up to us to help them.

Senator AKAKA. Thank you.

Secretary Juarbe and Admiral Cooper, describe how your agencies interact and communicate in working toward a goal of seamless transition.

Adm. COOPER. Let me discuss it from the VA side. The seamless transition, as I see it, first starts with those who are seriously disabled, and that is the reason we set up the special offices at both Walter Reed and Bethesda. These are the primary entry points for returning OEF/OIF servicemembers who are seriously disabled. We monitor them very carefully, as I said, so that if they are discharged, we can adjudicate their claims immediately. We also want to make sure we have all the medical records if they are discharged. So the primary point is to get every piece of information, talk to them, make ourselves available, and also be prepared once they are discharged. If they stay in the service, of course, we still communicate with them and advise them about the various services that are available while they are in the service.

When an individual leaves Walter Reed, Bethesda, or any of the other facilities where we have personnel stationed, we notify the VHA hospital and the regional office of jurisdiction in the area to which they are going.

The regional office will assign an individual to contact the veteran. VHA will receive the medical records and VBA will receive the necessary records for filing claims. We continue to communicate with individuals, particularly as regards vocational rehabilitation, to ensure that they know what benefits are available. If they decide to do nothing immediately, we have mandatory follow-ups at 6 months and 1 year to say, "OK, would you like to talk about it now? Is there something more we can do?"

So I think we have a pretty solid process in place.

Senator AKAKA. Thank you.

Secretary Juarbe?

Mr. JUARBE. Senator Akaka, there is obviously great need for coordination. Much is needed. And we do our part in working together both with the Department of Defense and with the Department of Veterans Affairs. We have a tremendous resource in our national network of local veterans employment representatives and Disabled Veterans Outreach Program specialists. DVOPs, the latter group, is one that works integrally with the Department of Veterans Affairs through their vocational rehabilitation and employment program. It may start with a referral, but then the referral back to them after the rehabilitation process has been completed and setting up a case management system for the individuals.

As I mentioned in my earlier statement, starting in November of 2003 we collaborated with the Departments of Defense and Department of Veterans Affairs and other partners at the State and private sector level to establish a recovery and employment assistance lifeline. With the establishing of the Joint Support Operations Center, we then felt that our program should work very closely with that center, and we are now integrally connected with them in that effort.

The importance is working with our partners at DOD and at VA, our focus on the earliest possible intervention and very personal services. Now, as Mr. Molino said, they are drinking from a fire hose at the very beginning with a considerable amount of information. But, Senator Akaka, this is one case where redundancy is desirable. We have heard this morning from the first panel that repetition is needed and frequency is needed. The important thing is timing and follow up.

The best way I can describe how some of that coordination can work effectively is a prime example that we have had with Sergeant Alfred Callas, who was featured in the GI Jobs issue this month, and I have a copy which I will make available to you. But in working with him as an amputee at Walter Reed, we have a representative located there, a Disabled Veterans Outreach Program specialist at Walter Reed who coordinated, identified what his interests were in employment upon returning home. And that is the key to following them up when they are back home.

He connected with the Disabled Veterans Outreach Program specialist in the State of Kansas, and eventually, because he was interested in going into a new field, that of auto mechanic and working on HMMWV, we were able to secure a job for him with Lear Siegler at Fort Riley, Kansas; in addition to that, working with the private sector. So what we did here is the Federal sector working together and working with the State sector, and then working with private industry, we were able to get Mack Tools to donate a set of tools for Sergeant Callas to enter into his new career.

That is how we see coordination, and that is a good example of how we see effective coordination from the earliest possible intervention all the way down to the home front.

Senator AKAKA. Admiral Cooper and Secretary Juarbe, are your employees in the trenches knowledgeable about the services that are offered by both VA and DOL so that they can give appropriate referrals to servicemembers, to agencies that they do not necessarily work for? For example, how are Disabled Veterans Outreach providers trained to appropriately refer veterans to agencies from which a veteran may benefit from utilizing services, specifically VA?

Admiral?

Adm. COOPER. I would say, yes, they are very well trained, especially in the Vocation Rehabilitation and Employment Program. This is an extremely well-run program. We did a study about a year-and-a-half ago to reorganize it and do everything we can to emphasize employment. When the young man or woman comes into our offices or comes into our program, we offer them options, or tracks, by which they can obtain employment, get an education, and/or become more independent in their daily living. I am firmly convinced that, although we need to continue training them, our VR&E counselors are well aware of the job opportunities, particularly in the areas where they are located and where they are helping veterans onsite.

Senator AKAKA. Secretary Juarbe.

Mr. JUARBE. Continued training is a key part of it, and we are focused through our National Veterans Training Institute, where our DVOPs and the LVERs are trained. We ensure that they are aware of the benefits and programs that are available through the Department of Veterans Affairs, and we work very closely with the Department of Veterans Affairs in the coordination of the DVOPs with the VR&E program, and providing briefings to the VR&E staff on USERRA issues and other employment issues.

Senator AKAKA. I have a question here from Senator Craig. As I mentioned earlier, he is unable to be with us at this moment because he has an amendment on the floor.

Senator Craig is impressed with the VA's program which wisely utilizes the talents of injured servicemembers like Mr. Wyatt. Are your departments doing anything similar to hire former servicemembers, Admiral?

Adm. COOPER. Yes. Our Department started the program that the Senator is talking about as an experiment. The CIO for VA began by hiring 9 or 10 returning veterans. In just the last 2 weeks this initiative has become a VA-wide program managed by the Office of Human Resources Management.

And I am also pleased that, in my own organization, the Veterans Benefit Administration, 47 percent of the personnel are veterans. The National Cemetery Administration is about 75 percent veterans. I think this demonstrates that VA is really trying to do everything they can.

Senator AKAKA. Secretary Molino?

Mr. MOLINO. Senator, the first thing you hear from an injured soldier is what you heard this morning. Their first desire is to stay on active duty, go back with their unit and serve with their colleagues. When we can, the services are committed to doing just that. There have been stories in the press about disabled servicemembers who are able to return to active duty, full active duty with their units. When that does not happen the services offer the opportunity to find employment as a career civil servant either with the same service with which the person is familiar or in the broader Department of Defense or even beyond the Department of Defense to other Government agencies.

We have two programs working within the Department of Defense to identify folks to take advantage of that. We are beginning with kind of an interim program where they can learn the skills, kind of try on the job and see if that is what they think they want to do with the rest of their lives. The Air Force indeed has a mandate that they have imposed upon themselves, if an Air Force airman is injured severely and cannot stay on active duty, they will find a job for that individual if they choose to take the job.

So, yes, we are very aggressively doing that. And as I said earlier, Senator, these are very talented young Americans and we do not want to lose them. If they cannot stay in uniform and continue to serve, we would welcome them as civilian employees.

Senator AKAKA. Secretary Juarbe.

Mr. JUARBE. The Veterans Employment and Training Service has the lead role in a program that is known as the Disabled Veterans Hiring Initiative, which is we have reached out to all Federal agencies, in partnership with the VA also, to talk about the special hiring authorities, the known competitive hiring authorities that are available to facilitate employment for disabled veterans, the severely disabled veterans. That is a program that we are very pleased with. In the Department of Labor, within my own Agency, we have a high level of veterans of course, and we are constantly looking for opportunities.

Senator AKAKA. Secretary Juarbe, I have two questions here from Senator Craig. How do you track DOL's efforts to provide employment assistance to recently separated combat veterans? Is priority given to these individuals? How many recently separated servicemembers who have sought DOL's employment assistance later found jobs?

Mr. JUARBE. The follow-up and tracking is an integral part of the services that are performed by the DVOPs and the LVERs, and at the One-Stop Career Centers our approach has always been focused on case management and follow-up. The reporting from veterans is controlled through the Employment and Training Administration reports that we get on the ETA 9002, which is the macro report for the public labor exchange services to veterans. From that we derive the information concerning the services that are provided by the Disabled Veterans Outreach Program specialists and the local veterans employment representatives under the VETS Form 200.

Through REALifelines we are also tracking those servicemembers who have elected to enroll in the program, and we are working together with the Joint Support Center to continue that tracking of those individuals. Under the REALifelines Program we have been able to track—we have been working with approximately 200 cases since we started the program last October, and about 15 percent of those have resolved and resulted in decisions regarding employment, training or other opportunity outcomes.

Senator AKAKA. Secretary Juarbe, this question is from Senator Craig. 1,700 Idahoans were deployed to Iraq last November as part of the 116th Brigade Combat Team. Your Agency has the oversight responsibility of the law guaranteeing reemployment rights upon their return home. The question is, what activities have you undertaken to prepare for the return of these guardsmen so that complaints are held to a minimum?

Mr. JUARBE. Since September 11, 2001 the Department of Labor, and through my agency, has had an aggressive compliance assistance outreach program, where we have provided briefings and technical assistance to over 240,000 individual members of the Guards and Reserves and employers. That outreach continues, and it has been in partnership with the U.S. Chamber of Commerce, the Society for Human Resource Management, the National Federation of Independent Businesses and other labor organizations like that and business organizations. And we provide pre-mobilization briefings and post-mobilization briefings.

As I stated in my statement earlier, we recognize that there is an increased need for providing transition assistance to these individuals, even though most of them ostensibly will be returning back to a job if they are members of the Guards and Reserves, and those rights are protected. We know that many of them may not have an interest in pursuing other career opportunities, and also for those where their jobs are no longer there because the company may have gone out of business.

What we have found is that as a result of this outreach we have been able to reduce the level of incidents of discrimination, and when those incidents of discrimination—and this is in comparison with the last major call-up of 265,000 in the Persian Gulf War. When we do address those incidents, with our partners, the Department of Defense National Committee on Employer Support of the Guard and Reserve which is our first line of defense out there with over 4,000 volunteers, is we are able to resolve many of these issues on an informal basis. Many employers simply did not understand the law, and they are willing to comply with it.

We determined from that that there was a need for regulations, and to that extent we published regulations last fall for comments and we hope to issue the final regulations on USERRA, which was enacted in 1994, but those regulations should be out some time this year.

We also have the poster which is now published and available for all employers who are supposed to make the information available through a poster or other means of the rights and responsibilities that individuals have under USERRA.

Senator AKAKA. My final question is to Admiral Cooper and Assistant Secretary Juarbe. We are anticipating a greater demand of Veterans Affairs as well as Department of Defense by our military people as well as our veterans, and we have been looking at our budget. So my question is on the budget to both of you. How have Veterans Affairs and Labor's budgets been increased to reflect the increased workload as a result of the present conflict? Admiral?

Adm. COOPER. Our budget has essentially increased probably about 2 to 3 percent. Also, you may remember, last year and the year before, Secretary Principi, through the Supplemental Appropriation, was able to give us some extra money, and last year, transferred funds from the VHA budget to VBA. This allowed us to use 75 million this year, and we will have 50 million extra in our budget this following year. So I would say those two are major moves that were made.

Mr. JUARBE. Each year during my tenure at the Veterans Employment and Training Service, we have had an increase in our budgets, and for fiscal year 2006 we do have another increase in the total funding. We will increase the Jobs for Veterans Act grants which fund the outreach personnel, the VET reps, or the DVOPs and LVERs at the State level, with an increase of $1.3 million. The services to homeless veterans also are being increased. That is a program that is increasing by $1.2 million for fiscal year 2006.

Senator AKAKA. I want to thank my panelists very much for your responses today.

It will, no question, be helpful to the Committee. There may be questions of Members. We would submit that for the record. We look forward to a better way of trying to service our veterans as well as our military personnel. I personally look forward to working with all of you in doing that, and by sharing information as we have we will be able to do that.

So with that, thank you very much for being here this morning. The hearing stands adjourned.

[Whereupon, at 11:48 a.m., the hearing was adjourned.]

APPENDIX

Question 1: If a recently separated National Guard member files a disability compensation claim for Post Traumatic Stress Disorder (PTSD), what priority is that claim given in the system? Do you believe all claims by recently separated combat veterans should be adjudicated on a priority basis?

Response: The Veterans Benefit Administration (VBA) is giving top priority to the benefit claims of all returning war veterans, including National Guard members, who have serious physical injuries, and providing the best possible service to these returning heroes must remain our highest priority. Claims from terminally ill veterans, homeless veterans, veterans with severe financial hardship, and former prisoners of war also receive priority attention.

Our goal must be to provide quality, timely, and compassionate service to all claimants. As a result, we do not believe that VA should adopt a policy of adjudicating all claims by recently separated combat veterans on a priority basis.

Question 2: Of all the servicemembers medically discharged from service in the last 3 years, how many converted their life insurance coverage from SGLI to VGLI? Isn't this the population that would have the most difficulty purchasing life insurance in the commercial market? What more can be done, either by VA or the Congress, to emphasize the importance of this transitional benefit?

Response: Medically discharged servicemembers need Veterans' Group Life Insurance (VGLI) most because the disabilities they incurred in service often make them uninsurable by private commercial companies unwilling to take a risk insuring an "unhealthy life."

We do not have specific information regarding the number of servicemembers medically discharged from service who converted their Servicemembers' Group Life Insurance (SGLI) to VGLI. However, we have information showing that, since June 2001, 51 percent of separating servicemembers with military disability ratings of 50 percent or higher have applied for VGLI.

The Department of Veterans Affairs (VA) and the Office of Servicemembers' Group Life Insurance (OSGLI) conduct extensive outreach to separating and recently separated members concerning VGLI. The outreach includes:

• Providing all separating servicemembers, as part of the transitional assistance program (TAP) and disabled transitional assistance program (DTAP) briefings, and informational brochures on VA insurance programs. The brochures describe the importance of insurance and also provide eligibility information and a VGLI application.

• Mailing VGLI applications to all separating servicemembers. OSGU sends all separating servicemembers VGLI applications to their address of record. A first mailing is sent 30 to 60 days after discharge; a second is sent if there is no response within 2 weeks to the first mailing, and a third is sent at the end of the 1-year and 120-day period in which to convert to VGLI.

• Conducting "special outreach" to the most disabled separating servicemembers. Specifically, the VA Insurance Service conducts computer matches to identify those servicemembers who have medically retired with a military disability rating of 50 percent or more who have not applied for VGLI or the SGU 1-year extension available to totally disabled servicemembers. These servicemembers are contacted by phone and provided assistance in applying for VA insurance, including VGLI and the SGLI extension.

Through this outreach effort, approximately 38 percent of those contacted convert their insurance coverage. Prior to our outreach, 20 percent or less converted their insurance coverage. To date, about $96 million in insurance has been granted as a result of these outreach efforts.

Question 3: I am impressed with your program, which wisely utilizes the talents of injured servicemembers like Tristan Wyatt. Are you aware of a larger Federal effort on this front, or is this program peculiar to VA?

Response: In 2001, VA established a national veterans' employment program to assist all veterans in understanding veteran's preference and in accessing information on job opportunities in VA and other Federal agencies. Under this initiative, VA has participated in job fairs and career conferences; developed a website for veterans; and distributed brochures, posters, and CD-ROMs to military transition centers around the country.

VA recently launched a nationwide initiative to assist injured and disabled servicemembers returning from Operations Enduring Freedom (OEF) and Operation Iraqi Freedom (OIF) in finding employment. The initiative will expand VA's Vet-information technology program, which provides volunteer work experience and employment to service-connected disabled veterans. Currently, efforts are underway to work with other Federal agencies, State and local officials, and private industry to provide job training, work experience, and career opportunities to medically discharged veterans.

Question 4: At our last hearing GAO testified about some of the circumstances where the transition between DOD care and VA care aren't working seamlessly. One of those mentioned was that VA has no policy for maintaining contact with those veterans who may need time to adjust to the idea that they are too disabled to continue their military career and need to prepare for civilian jobs, thus they do not apply immediately for VA's vocational rehabilitation services. Describe for me some of the successful ways that VA's regional offices maintain contact with these individuals. What are you doing to rectify the problem GAO identified?

Response: VBA released its first policy letter (20–03–36) to all field stations on September 23, 2003. That policy letter outlined procedures for outreach, coordination of VA services, and claims processing for OIF/OEF servicemembers and veterans.

VBA policy letter 20–05–14, dated March 8, 2005, updated and expanded outreach and claims processing procedures for serving OIF/OEF servicemembers and veterans. This letter was jointly developed by the VBA Office of Field Operations and the VBA business lines, including Vocational Rehabilitation and Employment (VR&E). It Outlines specific outreach and coordination of VA services. Regional office (RO) directors are responsible for ensuring that VA maintains contact with seriously wounded servicemembers. Some of the procedures outlined in the policy letter pertain to outreach conducted by the ROs and providing VR&E benefits and services. Those activities include:

• Each RO director must designate an OIF/OEF coordinator and an alternate.

• An OIF/OEF case manager is assigned for each compensation claim received from a seriously disabled OIF/OEF servicemember.

• Points-of-contact are established with military and VA medical facilities.

• Education about available VA benefits, including VR&E benefits, and delivery of these benefits are coordinated and claims are managed by a case manager.

• The RO director or assistant director must call returning seriously disabled servicemembers when they first arrive in the RO's jurisdiction to welcome them home and advise them that they will be contacted by the OIF/OEF coordinator.

Procedures in the national policy directive which specifically relate to VR&E include:

• After an entitlement disability has been established for an OIF/OEF servicemember, a VR&E counselor with jurisdiction over the hospital or medical holding company at a military facility will visit the servicemember to begin counseling and evaluation prior to discharge.

• If, after initial contact, the servicemember or veteran does not respond or indicates "no interest," VR&E will diary for a follow-up contact no later than 1 year after the initial contact.

• VR&E officers will ensure that an indicator is affixed to the Counseling/Evaluation/Rehabilitation folder identifying that the veteran served in OIF/OEF. VR&E will maintain a log of each of the OIF/OEF veterans they have contacted and with whom they are working.

Question 5: Also at last month's hearing, GAO mentioned the need for VA and DOD to reach a formal information-sharing agreement so that VA can have systematic access to DOD data about populations who need VA services. What specifics does this agreement need to have to make sure that VA can appropriately deliver services? What has been the holdup in reaching this agreement? How do you suggest we can help facilitate this agreement?

Response: VA's Office of General Counsel negotiated a memorandum of understanding (MOU) with the Department of Defense (DOD) to obtain the complete range of returning servicemember data VA needs for identification, tracking, and statistical/reporting purposes. This MOU addresses the transfer of information, including protected health information, on all servicemembers who are about to transition from DOD to VA or who are eligible for benefits administered by VA during their active duty. The MOU has been signed by VA officials and is with DOD for concurrence.

RESPONSE TO POST-HEARING QUESTIONS SUBMITTED BY HON. LARRY E. CRAIG, CHAIRMAN, TO JOHN M. MOLINO, DEPUTY UNDER SECRETARY OF DEFENSE FOR MILITARY COMMUNITY AND FAMILY POLICY, DEPARTMENT OF DEFENSE

Question 1: How many Federal agencies have a presence at military treatment facilities like Walter Reed? Is there a worry about overwhelming injured servicemembers with information? How have the Military Services coordinated the well-intentioned efforts of other agencies so that the information provided can be absorbed at the appropriate time and pace of the injured servicemember?

Answer: The presence of Federal agencies varies at military treatment facilities. For example, Walter Reed established a service delivery system, "TEAMS" (Transition Employment Assistance Management Services), to effectively coordinate both internal and external agencies' efforts to provide transition and employment assistance to servicemembers and their families at the appropriate time. This system includes the following:

DEPARTMENT OF VETERANS AFFAIRS (VA)

• VA Benefits Administration—to provide servicemembers comprehensive benefits counseling, assist in filing claims for VA benefits, obtain all relevant Army medical records, provide complete medical examinations, and process the VA applications for benefits, to include rating, prior to separation from active duty.

• VA Office of Information and Technology (OI&T)—established VET IT program designed to provide mentoring, coaching, and/or training to servicemembers in transition from military service to the civilian sector with the ultimate goal being employment within VA OI&T.

DEPARTMENT OF LABOR (DOL)

• DOL Employment & Training Service—facilitates Transition Assistance Program (TAP) consisting of instruction, information and assistance to members of the Armed Forces who are within 180 days of separation and their spouses in line with the mandates of 10 U.S.C. 1144.

• DOL Recovery and Employment Assistance Lifelines (REALifelines) Initiative established to ensure that wounded and injured servicemembers and their families get the support they need to be successful and competitive as they return to their homes by adding resources at the Federal, State, and local levels.

OFFICE OF PERSONNEL MANAGEMENT (OPM)

• OPM—A representative will be assigned to Walter Reed 2 days of the week to coordinate outreach activities with WRAMC TAP Staff and provide Federal employment information to servicemembers and family members; serve as point-of-contact for other Federal agencies interested in providing employment opportunities and job search assistance; encourage Federal agencies to identify and establish collaborative endeavors to meet servicemembers' transition and employment needs; provide Federal employment and education information; and, upon request, participate in activities that further support WRAMC TAP.

DEPARTMENT OF DEFENSE (DOD)

• Computer/Electronic Accommodation Program (CAP)—provides assistive technology for wounded servicemembers and employees with disabilities. The Defense Applicant Assistance Office (DAAO)—"Temporary Assignment Program" initiative supports servicemembers in acquiring new work experiences and skills; networking opportunities and resources through temporary Federal work assignments that may lead to Federal employment opportunities with participating Federal agencies upon servicemembers' separation.

ARMY CAREER ALUMNI PROGRAM (ACAP)

• Coordinates delivery of DOD Transition Assistance Program with TEAMS that empowers servicemembers to make informed career decisions through benefits counseling and employment assistance (including pre-separation briefings) and provides two employer databases of employers expressing interest in hiring servicemembers.

WRAMC has developed a Memorandum of Understanding with the Office of Personnel Management (OPM) that will allow, once implemented, OPM to set up a liaison office to coordinate with all other Federal agencies that want to interface with severely injured servicemembers. This workable arrangement came about as a result of an Employment Transition Summit hosted by WRAMC in January 2005, and participated in by DOD, the Military Services and Federal agencies.

Thanks to the establishment of the Military Severely Injured Center (a "24/7" call center staffed by nurses and master's level social workers), the Department is able to ensure the full scope of these services to each severely injured servicemember on a personal basis, when the servicemember is ready to absorb the information and make informed decisions.

Question 2: In order to ensure that no injured servicemember "falls through the cracks" when discharged, it is vital that DOD share with other Federal agencies the identities of these individuals. How is DOD working with VA and others on this front?

Answer: DOD established the Military Severely Injured Center on February 1, 2005, to supplement Military Service efforts and ensure all "seams and gaps" are filled. The Center is staffed with trained nurses, social workers, and VA, DOL and Transportation Security Administration representatives in a "24/7" call center to ensure the severely injured and their families receive the support and care they need. Counselor/Advocates with master's degrees in social work and nursing are also being located around the country near military treatment facilities, VA hospitals, and community-based hospitals to provide outreach support to severely injured and their families and to ensure coordination with the Center care managers and other Federal agencies, as necessary. The Center also serves as a backstop to support Military Services and other Federal agencies intended to help severely injured and their families if they hit a roadblock (whether medical care, finances, education, job assistance, counseling or transition issues) while on active duty or when they are discharged. DOD works directly with the VA and other Federal agencies (to include sharing identities of severely injured, as necessary and appropriate, protecting privacy, as required). The Center provides a "warm hand-off" and appropriate follow-up between agencies to ensure that no one "falls through the cracks." In addition to the Center, the program is supported by ten working groups, comprised of members of the DOD, Military Services and Federal agency staffs, that are responsible for extending support beyond the medical centers and defining solutions to difficult systemic issues that confront the severely injured and their families.

The Department of Defense is working with VA to provide information on OEF/OIF servicemembers.

- Recently Separated OEF/OIF Veterans-Active Duty and Reserve Components:
- The Defense Manpower Data Center (DMDC), on behalf of Health Affairs, began routinely providing VA rosters of OEF and OIF veterans who have separated from active duty in September 2003. In June 2004, DMDC instituted a new process that more accurately identified those who deployed to the OEF/OIF combat theaters. The accuracy of the DMDC OEF/OIF veteran rosters being provided today to VA is excellent. The DMDC rosters for the VA will continue to improve and will be regularly discussed by the DOD-VA Deployment Health Working Group.
- Active Duty Servicemembers in the Physical Evaluation Board/Medical Evaluation Board (PEB/MEB) Process:
- DOD has worked with VA to draft a Memorandum of Understanding that will ensure compliance with HIP AA as the two Departments share protected health information. The MOU is presently being staffed at VA for signature.
- The Office of the Assistant Secretary of Defense (Health Affairs), Clinical and Program Policy has drafted a policy to provide authority and guidance on how DOD will collect critical data elements on severely injured and ill soldiers and provide this information to the VA. Under this policy—Expediting Veterans Benefits to Members with Serious Injuries and Illnesses—DOD would transmit needed data to the VA "promptly, securely (virtual private network or secure system), and electronically from the Services, through Health Affairs, to the Department of Veterans Affairs."

RESPONSE TO POST-HEARING QUESTIONS SUBMITTED BY HON. LARRY E. CRAIG, CHAIRMAN, TO FREDERICO JUARBE, JR., ASSISTANT SECRETARY FOR VETERANS AND TRAINING, VETERANS EMPLOYMENT AND TRAINING SERVICE, DEPARTMENT OF LABOR

Question 1. How do you track DoL's efforts to provide employment assistance to recently separated combat veterans? Is priority given to these individual? How many recently separately servicemembers who have sought DoL's employment assistance later found jobs?

Answer. No answer submitted by time of press.

Question 2. 1,700 Idahoans were deployed to Iraq last November as part of the 116th Brigade Combat Team. Your agency has the oversight responsibility of the law guaranteeing re-employment rights upon their return home. What activities have you undertaken to prepare for the return of these Guardsmen so that complaints are held to a minimum?

Answer. No answer submitted by time of press.

Question 3. As the agency tasked with ensuring that veterans receive preference when competing for Federal employment, what efforts has the Department of Labor made to be a model employer of veterans? Does DoL have prgorams in place similar to VA's that seeks to employ recently separated veterans or seriously wounded veterans?

Answer. No answer submitted by time of press.

○